The Doctor's Guide

Science for a Healthy Life

Tyler Miksanek, MD

CONTENTS

CHAPTER 1: INTRODUCTION

WHY A VALLEY IN ECUADOR IS FILLED WITH AMERICAN RETIREES

For all its faults, modern medicine has come a long way. Sure, today's healthcare is often expensive, complicated, and impersonal. But our modern system remains a heck of a lot better than having the town doctor stick leeches on you and hoping for the best. Life expectancies have doubled in just a few generations, and new advances have turned diagnoses that were once death sentences into treatable conditions. Nonetheless, twenty-first century medicine would still fall head over heels for a fountain of youth, or some similar magic cure that could eliminate suffering and help us live longer. And surprisingly, not too long ago, researchers thought they were close to finding a modern fountain of youth deep in the heart of South America.

Located in the country of Ecuador, Vilcabamba is a small village nestled amid sloping coffee fields. Its tropical South American location, combined with an elevation almost a mile above sea level, means that the weather remains close to 70°F year round. The favorable climate, plus the high quality of the soil, fills the area with the bold greens of lush vegetation and the softer hues of centuries-old farms. Surrounded by dramatic, jagged mountain peaks, Vilcabamba truly resembles an idyllic fairytale village. Matching its enchanted appearance, Vilcabamba also has a magical-sounding claim to fame. Billing the town as being located in the 'Valley of Longevity,' locals boast that they frequently live to age 100 or older, unburdened by many of the chronic diseases and ails associated with aging.

So what contributes to the long lifespans of the Vilcabamba community? Is it the agreeable climate? The local diet? The pastoral lifestyle? Or were the locals simply the lucky recipients of favorable genes that granted them unnaturally good health? When researchers first descended into the Vilcabamba valley in the 1970s, these were the questions on their minds. Of course, being good scientists, they also had to treat locals' claims with a healthy dose of skepticism. On first glance, however, the village lived up to its reputation. Researchers found the locals to be much older on average than broader demographics at the time would predict, giving support to the idea that there was truly something special about Vilcabamba. Even more impressive, elderly locals were able to show researchers baptismal records, seemingly confirming their impressive ages. Imagine the shock of an outsider hearing a villager claim to be 122 years old, and then having an official document to prove it!

I first heard of the association between Vilcabamba and longevity as a college student studying abroad in Ecuador. Admittedly, I never gave it much thought until one day, on a hike not far from Vilcabamba, I came across two Americans on the trail. Mountainous and at an air-thinning 12,000 feet of elevation, the hike would have been strenuous for anyone. But seemingly confirming the local promises of impressive aging, these fellow hikers looked quite old. Curiosity got the best of me, and I awkwardly asked how two elderly Americans had ended up on a mountainside in rural Ecuador. Luckily, the hikers were quite friendly, and freely told me their story. They had been best friends for decades. Now, aged 78, they were both recently widowed, and had been stuck wondering what the next chapter of their lives would look like. They had heard of the region's pleasant climate and positive effects on health, and decided to make the move from the U.S. to Ecuador a few months prior. Thrilled with their decision, they had been travelling around the area and trying to do as much hiking as possible.

Watching them trek away along the challenging mountain trail, I stood awed at their physical endurance that seemed to openly defy their age. I could have been convinced right there and then that Vilcabamba truly did have some magic fountain of youth. After returning from the hike, I asked a friend from Ecuador for more information about Vilcabamba. She told me she too had recently visited, also intrigued by the claims of century-old Ecuadorean farmers still actively working their fields. But instead, she told me with a smile, "everyone there looks like you."

Her comment made me chuckle. Brown haired, blue eyed, and white, I fit the average description for the modern day inhabitants of what had become a thriving expatriate community. Instead of the elderly Ecuadorean locals that had fascinated researchers a generation earlier, Vilcabamba was now largely filled with retired Americans and Europeans hoping for continued good health in the famed Valley of Longevity. A quick online search showed page after page of expats writing glowing reviews of the weather, the scenery, and the relaxed pace of living. And on almost every page, the area's claim to long, healthy lives was highlighted. The area was certainly popular, but the claims to health seemed suspicious. Sure, the hikers I had seen on the mountain trail were in great shape, but they had only moved to the area several months prior. Regardless of the cause for the locals' longevity, I doubted a few months stay in Vilcabamba could magically rejuvenate American retirees.

It turns out, I was not the only one who was skeptical. Remember that local who had claimed to a visiting researcher that he was 122 years old? Three years later, when the researchers returned, the same man claimed to be 134. Something was amiss. Researchers turned to the baptismal records that villagers offered as proof of their ages. They quickly found that in such a small community, there were few family names, and many children were named after older relatives. As a result, many of the locals' names were the exact same. By asking for their godparents' names, also documented on the baptismal records, the researchers were able to determine that many of the villagers' claims did not stand up to further scrutiny. Instead of being their own birth records, the records often belonged to an older relative who shared the same name. Further work showed that locals frequently exaggerated their ages, likely to increase their standing in a community that valued the elderly. And while the proportion of elderly villagers in the community was higher than expected, the discrepancy could be explained by younger residents leaving to find work elsewhere, not the elderly living much longer than expected. In fact, the researchers concluded that average lifespan in Vilcabamba was actually 15 to 30% lower than in the U.S.

The story of Vilcabamba offers two important lessons

in analyzing claims about secrets to good health and longevity. First, it can be extremely difficult to discern if a claim really is too good to be true. Subpar research focusing on the skew toward an older population in Vilcabamba, coupled with locals' apparent proof of their ages through baptismal records, easily could have led to the incorrect conclusion. And second, just because a claim does not stand up to scrutiny does not mean that it will fail to gain widespread attention. After all, Vilcabamba became a popular expat community well after its claim to unusual life expectancy was debunked.

The rapid availability of information on the Internet has multiplied the number of similar claims we are exposed to on a daily basis. Take, for example, the health benefits of flossing. The American Dental Association recommends flossing once a day. Guidelines like this one are important in the medical community, as they mean that a group of experts have reviewed the topic thoroughly and agreed on an official recommendation. However, simple guidelines can muddy more complicated truths. Many studies have been done on the efficacy of flossing, with some evidence that flossing can reduce levels of gum inflammation. That being said, some researchers question the available evidence, going so far as to argue that daily flossing should not be recommended. On the other hand, some dentists argue flossing is even more important than brushing one's teeth. There is a surprising amount of controversy in the world of dental research, and a simple Internet search on flossing is unlikely to reveal the actual complexity behind the official recommendations.

In fact, that simple Internet search is more likely than not to turn up some questionable claims. Multiple sites posit that the mere act of flossing can add 6.4 years to your lifespan. Many of these sites link to each other as 'proof' of the claim, without specifically citing any original research. The origin of the claim seems to rest with a 1999 book called RealAge, which in turn cites a 1993 study from *The British Medical Journal.* That study, while published in a highly respected journal, simply found an association between poor dental hygiene and an increased risk for heart disease. However, such an association does not necessarily mean that deciding to floss will magically add six years to your life. People who floss are, on average, less likely to be overweight, less likely to abuse alcohol, and more likely to regularly see a doctor than people who do not floss. All these associations mean that although healthy people are more likely to floss, they are not necessarily healthy because they floss. It's just like the hikers I met near Vilcabamba. They were leading a healthy lifestyle and enjoying the climate of the region, but it was not the region itself that was making them healthy. If one of the hikers were crippled by a bad knee and unable to walk, they probably would not have left the United States in the first place, and I certainly would not have run into them on a difficult mountain trail.

I'll be honest. I don't floss regularly. But I am a doctor, and frequently have to distill complex and often conflicting health claims and data into general recommendations for my patients. A great example is the use of statins. Statins are a class of medications used to lower cholesterol levels, and they are some of the most frequently prescribed drugs in America. There is good reason for statins to be so popular, as study after study has shown that they can reduce deaths from heart attacks and strokes. If a doctor recommends that you start taking a statin, know that they do not just lower cholesterol, they can literally save lives.

Unfortunately, pretty much every medication has side effects, and statins are no exception. Perhaps the most common side effect of statins is that some people develop muscle pains while using them. Doctors generally respond to these side effects by decreasing the dose or switching to a different type of statin. Of course, both doctors and patients would prefer if the muscle aches did not occur to begin with. So, is there any way to prevent them? The answer, confusingly, depends on who you ask.

Let me explain. Some doctors tell patients to take a supplement called Coenzyme Q10 alongside their statin to help prevent the onset of muscle-related side effects. Several studies, admittedly with relatively small sample sizes, have shown that taking Coenzyme Q10 can help prevent muscle cramps caused by statins. But there is also plenty of evidence that Coenzyme Q10 is no better than a placebo. The official guidelines have come down against recommending Coenzyme Q10, with both the American College of Cardiology and the American Heart Association taking positions against it. Somewhat ironically, the statement by the American Heart Association against Coenzyme Q10 came out just weeks after their own scientific journal published a study arguing that it was, in fact, effective.

All this conflicting research puts doctors like me in a bind. The argument for prescribing patients Coenzyme Q10 is simple. It very well might work for some patients, and even if it is just a placebo, it is unlikely to do much harm. But in recommending the supplement to my patients, I would be going against the recommendation of specialists. Patients could very easily lose their trust in my recommendations if they look up their new pill and find out that it is controversial, and patients might be angry that I'm asking them to spend money on a supplement that might not be doing anything at all. Worse, some of my patients use many medications daily, and adding even one more thing to take might complicate their medication regimen just enough that they forget to take another, much more crucial pill.

In an ideal world, I think many patients would prefer for their doctors to explain the pros and cons of controversial supplements like Coenzyme Q10, so that they can have a role in the decision making process. Us doctors call these conversations 'shared decision making,' and we are trained to involve patients in decisions whenever we can. But remember, Coenzyme Q10 is just one possible way to avoid one possible side effect of a statin. Statins have also been linked to liver damage, an increased chance of developing diabetes, and negative cognitive effects. Remember, these are great drugs, and plenty of high-quality studies have shown that they do much more good than harm. With the limited time I have during an appointment, I have to decide what information I want to discuss. Do I focus on the mixed data behind Coenzyme Q10? Should I acknowledge the theoretical risk of developing diabetes with statins? Or, more practically, should I talk about the bloodwork they should get after starting this new medication? Of course, any time I spend discussing statins takes away from other complaints my patients might have. Should I also try to discuss the rash they wanted me to look at? Or, do I use the remaining time to examine that pinching pain in their shoulder? Shared decision making takes time, and the complexity of many medical decisions complicates a doctor's ability to fully inform our patients during a short office visit.

Even within the rarified pages of medical journals, where there is plenty of space for leading researchers to explain their data, there is a lot conflicting information out there. And for every patient who wants to talk about the relative risks and benefits of each medication they are on, there is another patient who just wants to be told what is 'best.' But, as I have discussed with the mixed evidence behind flossing and Coenzyme Q10, the best option is not always clear.

There are two takeaways I want readers to get from this book. The first takeaway is what I have been demonstrating so far – the idea that good science is hard. Really hard. Hard to perform, hard to interpret, and hard to act on. So when you hear bold claims about near-immortal villagers, instant steps to add years to your life, or miracle drugs without side effects, remember that the truth is often more complicated than it first appears. The second takeaway is more subtle. It is the idea that even though it seems easy to throw up our hands and quit when research gives us headaches and contradictions, we can still use science and medicine to vastly improve the world around us. Quality science and attention to detail helped solve the tall tales of Vilcabamba. Flossing may be surprisingly controversial, but improvements in dental care over the last 100 years mean that your sore tooth is unlikely to kill you. And while statins do have side effects, they have also saved countless lives in the last few decades alone. At any moment, thousands of researchers and scientists are trying to learn more about how we can best lead long, healthy, and happy lives, and there is plenty to learn from their discoveries. Let's explore!

CHAPTER 2: DIET AND NUTRITION

WHY LOSING WEIGHT IS ONLY HALF THE BATTLE

Deep into my fourth year of medical school, mere months away from graduation, I found myself in clinic with a patient who had been struggling with weight gain. He had been reading about different diets online, and wanted to know what I thought about intermittent fasting as a method to lose weight. In the months before, I had delivered a baby and watched it take its first breath, sewn up a patient after a brutal 12 hour surgery, and done multiple rounds of CPR on a pulseless patient until successfully restoring a normal heartbeat. But I did not, as I sheepishly admitted to the man in front of me, know anything about the data behind intermittent fasting.

It has become a rather open secret that most American doctors learn shamefully little about diet and nutrition in medical school. A report on education in US medical schools found that, over four years of schooling, doctors-to-be averaged only 19 hours learning about nutrition. Several medical schools did not have any required nutritional education at all. Doctors often bemoan when patients do a quick online search of some medical topic. But maybe us doctors need to do more worrying about our own cursory education on nutrition. When researchers surveyed 646 cardiologists, only 8% claimed to have 'expert' knowledge on nutrition, although a whopping 95% said that they needed to give nutrition information and guidance as part of their practice. Patients are turning to their doctors as trusted sources of information on diet and nutrition, but receiving inexpert opinions.

Doctors do not just struggle with limited knowledge of nutrition, we also seem to struggle with following basic nutrition recommendations ourselves. That same survey found that only 20% of cardiologists reported eating at least five servings of fruit and vegetables every day, a classic dietary recommendation. I have lost track of how many times I have seen doctors and nurses counsel patients on healthy eating, then return to snacking on their potato chips or seeking out a donut.

Of course, medical professionals are not alone in eating an unhealthy diet. After all, more than 40% of Americans are obese, with obesity rates rising every year. Obesity puts a huge strain on the nation's healthcare dollars, costing around $150 billion yearly. And increasingly, obesity starts young, with about one in five American children now categorized as obese.

Why is obesity so common? The easy answer is that we have access to calories at a rate never before seen in human history. Our ancestors dealt with regular famines and often had to worry about storing enough food for winter. Even in wealthy countries like France and England during the Industrial

Revolution, estimates show that the poor only consumed about 1400 calories a day. Today, that amount of calories can easily be consumed in one single fast food meal.

Sure, the Industrial Revolution was a long time ago. But our relationship with food has also dramatically changed over just the last few generations. Americans in 1960 spent close to 20% of their paychecks on food. Now, food expenditures represent less than 10% of income, even as Americans spend more on restaurants and takeout. A dozen eggs in 1919 cost, completely unadjusted for inflation and rising incomes, about 62 cents on average. Sure, eggs are more expensive today, but remember that incomes have risen roughly 2000% over the last century. If the price of eggs would have kept pace with income, a dozen eggs would cost around $12.

Just as food has become cheaper, it has also become both easier to find and less healthy. 100 years ago, baking a pie would be an all-day affair, likely done from scratch in a home kitchen and saved for a special occasion. Now, I can pick up a premade pie at the grocery store whenever I want for about $10. Preservatives and additives have become increasingly common as the gap between food producers and consumers has widened. Fast food has transitioned from a rare treat to a national pastime. Research shows that even healthy plants and vegetables have become less nutritious in recent years, likely due to growers focusing on crop yield, not nutrition. Scarier still, this phenomenon of nutrient depletion may worsen with changing climate conditions over the next century.

The solution to America's obesity epidemic seems obvious. We need to eat less food, and the food we do eat needs to be healthier. Of course, this is easier said than done. Our brains adapted for a hunter-gatherer lifestyle where one's next meal was not guaranteed. As such, our bodies fear the threat of starvation more than the threat of obesity, and we are quite happy eating much more fat and sugar than we actually need to survive. Diets are hard to start, and notoriously hard to maintain, which is why doctors need to be better prepared for dietary questions, including whether intermittent fasting can help a patient lose weight.

So, how should I have best advised my patient? Is intermittent fasting a good weight loss solution? In order to answer the question, we should define exactly what intermittent fasting is. More traditional diets focus on telling you what you cannot eat. Intermittent fasting, on the other hand, lets you eat whatever you want. It just constrains when you can eat it. For example, intermittent fasters might eat unlimited calories from 4PM to 10PM, but then refrain from eating at all until 4PM the next day. Other intermittent fasters might pick a day of the week to fast completely. Studies show that intermittent fasting does work to help people lose weight, and some researchers have found that people lose roughly the same amount of weight through intermittent fasting as they do with traditional diets focused on cutting calories. Other studies, although largely performed in mice and not in humans, show that the intermittent fasting approach can reduce inflammatory markers in the blood, and could possibly decrease the risk of cancer while increasing life expectancy.

That information makes it sound like we should all start intermittent fasting. But there are a few important caveats. First, just because something makes a mouse live longer does not mean that it will make a human live longer. Also, excess weight has long been associated with increased rates of cancer and decreased life expectancy, so the benefits seen in mouse studies could just be from weight loss in general, not anything special about intermittent fasting. But perhaps most importantly, researchers can force their mice to practice intermittent fasting by controlling when the mice are given food. Unlike mice in a cage, hungry humans tired of intermittent fasting can just head to the kitchen and eat whenever they want. It turns out, the hardest thing about intermittent fasting is actually sticking to the schedule. Not eating for the vast majority of the day, or sometimes even for the entire day, is an extraordinarily difficult habit to keep. When researchers studied a group of patients who simply tried to cut calories, 68% were able to stick to the diet. But for the group of patients who tried intermittent fasting, only 29% could maintain their fasting schedule.

The difficulty of sticking with any diet strategy underlies most research on dieting and nutrition. It turns out that losing weight with a diet is not that hard to do. If you start eating less calories, either through eating less food or healthier food, you are likely to lose some weight. That is why people keep turning to fad diets – they work. I could tell all my overweight patients eating 2,500 calories a day to change their diet to 2,000 calories a day of dog food. If they stuck with the diet, they would certainly lose weight. But I would bet good money that no matter how efficacious the diet was, not many people would keep it up for long.

A classic debate in the dieting world is whether it is better to cut carbs or to cut fat. Research shows that, on average, people tend to lose weight faster with a low-carb diet than a low-fat diet. People following low-carb diets also tend to have better cholesterol and triglyceride numbers on bloodwork than their counterparts on low-fat diets. However, most of these findings are from short-term follow up visits, generally a few months after the diet began. Across multiple studies, when researchers check back with participants a full year later, they find no significant difference in weight loss between the low-carb group and the low-fat group. Again, it seems that the specific diet does not really matter. Instead, what matters is the ability to maintain the diet over time. And maintaining a diet, as anyone who has tried it can attest, can be extremely difficult. For this reason, study after study shows a relatively depressing trend with weight loss. People pick a diet and start it, and generally have some initial success in losing weight. But over time, people tend to revert to their old ways of eating, and the weight comes back on. In other words, diets help people lose weight, but they do not help people keep the weight off. This pattern is seen across age, gender, and socioeconomic status. So if you have ever struggled with sticking to a diet or keeping weight off, know that you are far from alone.

In 2001, a group of researchers planned a study to see if they could help people maintain healthy eating strategies for the long term. They titled their study Look AHEAD (short for 'Action for HEAlth in Diabetes' – scientists love their clever titles) and recruited over 5,000 participants. Half the participants were treated as a control group, and given standard counseling on diet, exercise, and weight loss. The other half were given an 'intensive lifestyle intervention,' which basically meant free access to pretty much anything the researchers thought could help them lose weight. They had weekly group visits to incentivize healthy eating and exercise, a personal counselor to help them meet their lifestyle goals, and were strongly encouraged to work out at least 175 minutes a week. If they desired it, members of this group were given free nutritional shakes as meal replacements to encourage calorie control and healthy eating. For anyone who had trouble losing weight, the program would pay for free, healthy meals and cooking classes. Participants struggling to lose weight could also be provided with weight loss medication.

The Look AHEAD trial continued for a decade, with researchers examining both weight loss and serious medical events (like heart attacks and strokes) in each group. At the end of the study, researchers looked at the percent of total body weight that members of each group had lost. The control group lost 3.5% of their total body weight on average. In comparison, the intensive lifestyle intervention group averaged a 6.0% total body weight loss.

So, did the intensive intervention work? The answer, like so many things in science, is complicated. Compared to the control group, the group given a wide array of weight loss resources lost almost twice as much weight on average. Presenting the findings using that comparison makes the intervention sound like a huge success. That being said, the difference between 3.5% and 6.0% total body weight loss ended up only being about six pounds. Now, six pounds of weight loss sounds like a great start to a diet, but it makes for a rather uninspiring finding after a decade-long research study. And remember, the researchers were not just looking at weight loss. They were also measuring complications of obesity. To do so, they counted the number of heart attacks, strokes, hospital admissions for chest pain, and deaths in each group. And despite the incredible array of resources offered in the study, there were no significant differences in these outcomes, even after a decade of follow up.

Focusing on this finding makes it seem like weight loss is futile. After all, a bunch of really smart researchers spent a lot of money on a decade-long program designed to help motivated participants lose weight. But at the end of a decade, all their interventions only helped people lose about six extra pounds. Even worse, that marginal extra weight loss failed to stop people from having less heart attacks and strokes.

However, not all the conclusions from the study were so gloomy. There were plenty of positive findings from the Look AHEAD study as well. Members of the intensive lifestyle intervention group were found to have better cholesterol levels, improved insulin sensitivity, less kidney disease, less diabetes medications, and improved quality of life when compared against the control group. They were also less likely to need hospitalization, and over the decade spent $5,280 less on healthcare expenditures. Sure, the Look AHEAD study could not find a huge difference in the number of heart attacks and strokes between the two groups during the study, but the intensive lifestyle intervention group sure looked healthier after the ten years were complete.

Interpreted this way, the Look AHEAD study is an incredible argument for the power of lifestyle interventions. The intensive lifestyle intervention group may have only lost six extra pounds on average, but even that small difference, over ten years, was enough to make them demonstrably healthier by the end of the study. We too often view lifestyle interventions, especially diets, as short-term fixes. Following this routine, many of my patients go on a diet for a month to lose ten pounds, only to find themselves regaining the weight not long after. The Look AHEAD study instead challenges us to think incredibly long term. Even after a decade, the risk of heart attacks and strokes barely budged for members of the intensive intervention group. But at the same time, they were noticeably healthier than the control group when researchers dived a little deeper. Maybe if the study had continued for a second decade or longer, researchers might have found bigger differences in mortality.

Other research agrees with these conclusions. The United States Preventive Services Taskforce conducted a systematic review of studies examining the effects of dietary interventions on mortality. These studies had follow up periods ranging from 3 to 15 years, and all of them failed to show a difference in mortality between their intervention and control groups. However, the same body of evidence also showed that individuals who underwent lifestyle interventions tended to have better blood pressure and cholesterol measurements, likely lowering their cardiovascular risk over many decades.

Even modern weight loss drugs face the same problems. Medications like Wegovy, Ozempic, Zepbound, and Mounjaro have made headlines in recent years for their ability to help people shed pounds quickly. The science behind them is extraordinarily impressive, with patients losing 15 to 20 percent of their total body weight while taking these medications. That level of weight loss is roughly three times the weight loss seen even in the intensive intervention group from the Look AHEAD trial, which was conducted before these newer medications were approved. But once patients stop taking the medications, they tend to gain the majority of the weight back in just a few short months.

The takeaway here is that a one month diet to lose weight is a short-term fix that is unlikely to have long-term effects on our health. We would better support our wellbeing by focusing on the long-term consequences of our dietary choices. Instead of cutting out dessert to lose ten pounds, and then gaining the weight back once we stop our diet, the weight loss evidence directs us to make lasting, durable changes to what we consume.

Durable changes, unfortunately, are easier said than done. People who could cut out salty snacks for a month would balk at the idea of never eating chips again. For this reason, I find that patients with hard and fast rules about what they can and cannot eat often struggle with keeping weight off.

Eventually, the cravings build up, causing them to revert to their old eating habits. So what are the characteristics of people who can actually stick to a diet and maintain their weight loss? People who keep healthy foods at home, increase vegetable intake, and who can cut out frequent consumption of sugary, fatty foods are more likely to keep weight down long term. In practice, this means making conscious decisions about what food to buy at the grocery store, as well as being realistic with our expectations about how big of changes we can make. Instead of vowing to cut out all snacks, I tend to recommend patients try keeping healthy snack options at home to satisfy their inevitable cravings. Instead of never having dessert, I suggest occasionally substituting fruit or other lighter options. And just as importantly, we need to remember that the occasional sumptuous burger or heaping bowl of ice cream does not mean our strides towards a healthier lifestyle are ruined. Lifestyle risks build up over years. One cheat day does not need to negate a healthy trend.

This advice sounds powerful, but it is also a little nonspecific. For some, the concept that all diets can be efficacious is liberating. But other people are looking for somewhat more concrete guidance. I think this desire for specific advice is what leads many physicians to discuss the Mediterranean diet with their patients. The Mediterranean diet is loosely defined, but most descriptions include high consumption of vegetables, fruits, nuts, and olive oil, comparatively smaller amounts of fish and dairy, and very limited red meat. Sugary, fatty, processed snacks are strongly discouraged. The Mediterranean diet has been linked to improved cardiovascular outcomes and decreased risk of everything from diabetes to cancer. It is a great starting ground for people looking for healthy eating inspiration. And most importantly, it can be staggeringly effective. One group of researchers estimates that by switching out their unhealthy American diets for the ideal Mediterranean diet, people could add over ten years to their life expectancy.

At the same time, traditional Mediterranean foods are not the only healthy foods out there, and one reason why the Mediterranean diet is so frequently discussed is simply because it has been so well studied. Beyond the Mediterranean diet, there is a whole world of healthy, delicious food. Cucumbers, cherries, and walnuts all originated from Asia. Peppers, squash, and cashews are all from the Americas. Artichokes, okra, and watermelon hail from Africa. Plenty of cultures have created healthy, flavorful dishes. Our problem is that modern American cuisine, while delicious, relies too heavily on red meat, simple starches, and processed foods full of sugar and fat. Our brains, designed to survive the winter, not worry about diabetes, eat it all up. But luckily, small dietary changes, as long as they are maintained for the long haul, have been shown to have immense power in letting us live longer, healthier lives. The study estimating life expectancy gains from a complete switch to the Mediterranean diet also found that people would still increase their longevity with more modest dietary substitutions. In other words, we do not necessarily need to overhaul our eating to drastically improve our health. Small changes work wonders as well.

What are good ways you can start these changes? For most of us, food decisions for the week start at the grocery store. Prune your shopping list of some unhealthy snacks and desserts, and make a conscious decision to limit impulse purchases while at the store. By having healthier food at home in the first place, we set ourselves up for success. If you are eating red meat two or three times a week, try to cut it down to one or two. If you find yourself snacking on sugary or salty snacks late at night, try replacing unhealthy snacks with a healthier alternative like crunchy vegetables or a cup of herbal tea. If you find yourself drinking lots of calories through sodas and juices, find lower calorie alternatives.

If you want, you can drop your current diet right now and make a complete switch to the Mediterranean diet. But not everyone is ready or able to make and maintain such drastic changes. And as we have learned, the most important component of a diet is sticking with it. So I challenge you, pick a few dietary changes you can make today that you think you can sustain long term. After all, healthy eating is a lifelong adventure.

CHAPTER 3: EXERCISE

WHY THAT TREADMILL WON'T HELP YOU LOSE WEIGHT

A fit, toned body is just a few monthly payments away. At least, that is the message we receive in advertisements for gyms, where smiling, muscular actors without an ounce of body fat alternate between running effortlessly on treadmills and lifting weights. Other commercials, targeted towards those of us who would prefer to work out at home, make it seem like one elliptical or stationary bike is the only thing separating us from our skinniest selves. And yet, for all these claims of easy weight loss through exercise, I have lost count of how many patients I have talked to with the same fitness complaint. Some bought a new treadmill and have been using it every day. Others decided to jog two miles in the park before work each morning. A few dished out money for a pricey gym membership. They are all exercising regularly, they make sure to point out, but they are not losing any weight.

We have been trained to connect exercise with weight loss. But, believe it or not, exercise is actually a pretty poor way to lose weight. Contrary to what all those gym advertisements might make you think, working out is not the body's main way of burning calories. Instead, we burn the majority of the calories we consume simply through maintaining our basic vital functions. The body is constantly busy regulating our internal temperature, pumping our blood against gravity, and moving our muscles just to keep us breathing. All that work, which the body must do every second of every day, burns a lot more calories than a half-hour jog. In fact, studies estimate that roughly 60 to 70% of our total daily energy consumption is spent on these rudimentary, life-sustaining tasks. Everything else, including activity as simple as walking around our homes or moving our lips to chat with a friend, comes from the remaining 30 to 40% of our energy expenditure. So, even when we think we are drastically increasing the number of calories we burn through exercise, we end up making a much smaller difference in our total calorie consumption than we expect. The speed at which we burn calories on basic body functions, frequently referred to as our basal metabolic rate, can have a much greater effect on weight than how frequently we work out. People with a high basal metabolic rate can sit around and stay skinny, while people with low basal metabolic rates can gain weight even with regular exercise.

Adding insult to injury, exercise also encourages us to engage in what scientists call 'compensatory responses.' After people exercise, they tend to compensate by eating more food and doing less physical activity for the rest of the day, partially negating the benefits of their workout. Picture a man with a new exercise goal of running 30 minutes each morning. He goes on his run and burns 300 calories, feeling proud of himself for the accomplishment. But after his run, he is hungrier than normal, so he eats a bigger breakfast and lunch, ingesting 200 more calories than he usually does. Later in the day, he is still tired from his run and decides to watch TV when he would normally have done some light housework. If he would have burned 100 calories doing those household chores, his total energy balance for the day would be completely unchanged, even though he added a run to his routine. This pattern of us compensating for exercise shows up repeatedly in the scientific literature, with individuals losing less weight than expected.

In fact, using an exercise-only approach, many individuals fail to lose any weight at all. Expected weight loss from adding additional aerobic exercise to one's daily routine is just zero to three percent of total body weight. In other words, a 200 pound individual who starts an exercise program would expect to lose a maximum of 6 pounds. More significant weight loss can be seen with increased exercise duration, but the typical 30 to 60 minute daily exercise regimen tends to produce rather mediocre results.

So, how should people go about losing weight? It turns out that our diet has a much bigger impact on weight than exercise does. Multiple studies have compared weight loss achieved through dietary changes alone against weight loss from a combination of dietary changes and exercise. In these studies, exercise did seem to augment weight loss by a couple pounds, but the majority of the total weight loss could be achieved by dieting alone.

These studies should not be taken to mean that exercise is worthless. On the contrary, regular exercise has been associated with an incredible array of health benefits. A decreased risk of heart attacks, a smaller risk of developing cancer, improvements in blood pressure, and even a decreased risk of depression are all associated with regular exercise. Most importantly, routine exercise and increased physical fitness have been linked to decreased mortality. To put it simply, we should exercise not to lose weight, but because it helps us live longer. As a culture, we too often conceptualize exercise as a formal part of our day set aside to help us lose weight. Advertisements for gyms and treadmills can be quite catchy, hooking prospective customers in with promises of shedding pounds. But the truth is that while exercise is an imperfect weight loss tool, it is a great way to stay healthy.

I actually try to stay away from discussing 'exercise' with patients. For many people, the word itself conjures up failed experiments with dusty stationary bikes or unused gym memberships. Our fitness-obsessed culture often makes these very traditional forms of working out come to mind when people discuss exercise. Instead, I prefer to discuss 'physical activity.' After all, the idea that exercise has to be done in a gym or as a designated workout during the day narrows our opportunities to live an active lifestyle. Recognizing that physical activity is not limited to our stereotypes of exercise can be empowering. The middle-aged woman who cannot stand exercising after work on her treadmill probably loved the physical activity she had every day at recess back when she was in elementary school. Admittedly, we all outgrow the monkey bars, but similar to school aged children flocking to the playground, I challenge my patients to find small opportunities during the day to incorporate fun forms of physical activity. Even short bouts of exercise consisting of as little as 5 minutes of moderate activity at a time have been linked to longer lifespans. Starting a home improvement project, gardening in the backyard, or strolling a local museum are not necessarily what people traditionally think of as exercise, but they definitely involve more physical activity than watching TV.

While any movement is better than nothing, more intense forms of physical activity likely confer larger benefits over a shorter time period. But even these workouts do not need to look like the exercise stereotypes of people sweating at the gym. A tennis racket and balls can be bought for less than $20, and offer a fun, social way to burn calories quickly. Instructional dance videos online can be followed alone or with a partner, leading to a great indoor workout without spending a dime.

The lesson here is twofold. First, even without the large amounts of weight loss that people expect, there are real rewards to maintaining an active lifestyle. And second, with a little creativity and exploration, physical activity can and should be fun. Of course, even when people enjoy their exercise routine, finding time for a workout can still prove difficult. This dilemma leads many of my patients to ask exactly how much physical activity they need to do.

Luckily, there is some good research to follow here. Scientists working for the U.S. Department of Health and Human Services compiled official exercise guidelines, published in a report titled The Physical Activity Guidelines for Americans. These guidelines suggest that adults should perform at least 150 to 300 minutes a week of moderate-intensity physical activity. Moderate-intensity activities include brisk walking, yardwork such as raking leaves, or a casual bike ride. As defined by the guidelines, these activities are intense enough that they can make you break a sweat, but not so intense that they would stop you from talking while doing them. For busier individuals, the guidelines state that the same health benefits can be obtained from doing 75 to 150 minutes a week of vigorous-intensity activities. These activities, like running or high-speed biking, would generally make people too out of breath to hold a casual conversation. In addition to the recommendation for either moderate or vigorous activity, the guidelines also recommend that Americans do muscle-strengthening activities twice a week.

Personally, I view these guidelines as completely manageable. Following their definition, all it takes to be a healthy, active individual is a half hour of moderate activity five times a week, plus lifting some weights. And yet, less than 25% of Americans would meet these activity recommendations. As a country, we have some serious work to do.

Since the guidelines themselves are relatively modest, there are also people who argue more activity is better. Picture that ripped neighbor who gets up at 4AM to do a five mile run every day, only to hit the gym for a couple hours later in the afternoon. Unlike the average American, they are clearly going far and beyond our government's guidelines. Are we cheating ourselves out of potential health benefits by focusing on the government's exercise recommendations?

When researchers examined physical activity levels and mortality data from over half a million individuals, they found that increasing physical activity past the minimum recommended by the guidelines did in fact lower mortality even further. However, the extra gains were modest at best. Compared to individuals who reported performing no physical activity whatsoever, individuals who reported any activity at all were 20% less likely to die during the study's follow up period. Individuals who met the minimum amount of activity recommended by the guidelines were 31% less likely to die than their sedentary counterparts. Individuals doing a whopping three to five times the minimum, fitting the mold of our workaholic neighbor from the example above, were 39% less likely to die. So more activity definitely is better, but the biggest benefit comes from relatively small activity increases. Furthering this argument, a separate study showed that individuals who walked just 15 minutes a day, well below the recommended minimum activity levels, were 14% less likely to die than their inactive counterparts. Every additional 15 minutes of daily exercise lowered the risk of dying by four percent more.

There does seem to be an upper limit to the life-extending properties of exercise. That first study also looked at a select few super exercisers. These individuals reported doing at least ten times the recommended minimum levels of exercise. That amounts to 750 minutes of vigorous activity over the course of a week, more than twelve hours! But despite all of this exercise, they were no less likely to die than individuals who merely met the basic recommendations to qualify as active. Another study on joggers actually found an increased risk of death for individuals with the highest jogging intensity. Physical activity does wonders, but the benefits are not endless. In fact, most people can reap the vast majority of its benefits without a major time commitment. If you want to wake up for that 4AM run, be my guest. But sleeping in a bit longer will not prevent you from getting all the exercise you need.

In recent years, some fitness enthusiasts have actually questioned the need for that 4AM run. Most of the aerobic activity discussed so far falls under the umbrella of what exercise researchers would call moderate-intensity continuous training. In other words, the activity is done at a fixed level for a relatively long period of time, such as jogging at the same pace for a half hour. Some studies, however, have shown that high-intensity interval training, commonly abbreviated HIIT, may be a more efficient form of activity. HIIT workouts involve short bursts of intense activity, followed by cooldowns. So instead of running at a consistent pace, picture an all-out sprint for one minute, and then a period of walking before sprinting again. HIIT workouts are one of the few fads with a solid research base, as HIIT-inspired activity regimens have been shown to have increased benefits when compared against more traditional continuous training. And because of their focus on intense bursts of energy, HIIT workouts can allow people to reap the benefits of physical activity while spending less total time exercising. As with anything else, HIIT programs have their strengths and weaknesses. For busy people chronically crunched for time, they can serve as a way to make exercise as efficient as possible. However, the heavily-structured, intense nature of HIIT regimens might make them less appealing to individuals using physical activity as a way to destress.

Regardless of how it is structured, it is clear that aerobic exercise can quite literally add years to your life. But notice that cardio is not the only component of the government's physical activity guidelines, which also recommend two days a week of strength training. It is pretty easy to understand why giving the heart a workout with cardio might increase cardiovascular fitness, thereby helping us live longer. But the common perception of strength training is muscled men pumping iron in the gym, then admiring their chiseled reflections in the mirror. Are big biceps really that important to health? What is the evidence here?

I should clarify a bit. When the guidelines recommend two days a week of muscle-strengthening activities for adults, they are not asking an 85 year-old grandmother to start deadlifting in the gym. Younger adults might benefit most from lifting weights or completing stereotypical muscle-building activities like push-ups or sit-ups. In middle age, however, muscle-strengthening activities might transition to exercises like yoga or resistance band training. Most grandmothers would probably avoid weightlifting, but the elderly can still challenge their muscles through age-appropriate activities like gardening.

Regardless of one's age, there does seem to be a connection between muscle-building activities and mortality. Researchers used data from the U.K. to examine mortality rates in individuals who met the guideline recommendations for either muscle-building activity or aerobic activity, but not necessarily both. While the largest mortality benefit was observed in individuals who followed the guidelines for both muscle-building and aerobic activity, individuals who only met the minimum recommendations for muscle-building activity still had a decreased risk of dying.

Now, this sort of study design does not prove that strength exercises alone actually decrease mortality. The same results would be obtained if healthy people were simply more likely to do muscle-building exercises in the first place, even if their muscle training was not the thing making them healthy. Strong people tend to live longer, but that does not necessarily mean that lifting a few weights will greatly improve just anyone's health. In fact, when elderly women were randomized to either participate in a strength-training exercise program or serve as an inactive control group, researchers did not find any difference in outcomes such as fracture risk or cognitive function after a three year follow up. However, drawing extensive conclusions from this one study may be unfair. After all, we know that strength training helps build muscle while burning fat. While this exchange might not lead to overall weight loss or magically keep the brain young, these changes to our body composition can still make us healthier overall. Many studies back this argument up, showing that individuals randomized to strength training end up with lower blood pressure and less risk of diabetes.

The concept that we can have a healthier body composition without necessarily losing weight is an important one. Doctors have long classified people into being underweight, normal weight, overweight, or obese by calculating a body mass index, or BMI. The BMI calculation is a pretty simple one: take weight and divide by height squared. Using BMI has both strengths and weaknesses. One strength of BMI is its simplicity, as measuring height and weight at a physician's office or at home takes only seconds. But BMI is also used because it correlates with health outcomes in study after study. BMIs in the normal weight category are associated with the longest lifespans. As BMI increases and individuals move from overweight to obese, mortality rates increase with each extra pound. We are literally talking about years of life here, as a 40 year old with a normal BMI is predicted to live about four years longer than a 40 year old categorized as obese.

The main downside of BMI is that by only taking weight and height into account, it is a rather simplistic definition of physical fitness. Remember our 4AM runner from earlier? Imagine that all the hours our runner puts in at the gym has allowed them to bulk up on muscle mass. The scale cannot tell the difference between muscle and fat, meaning that those extra pounds from muscle gain show up in the BMI calculation. For this reason, many muscular athletes can be overweight or even obese using BMI, even if they barely have any body fat at all. Some researchers have noted that the relationship between BMI and mortality is less obvious if one controls for other measures of physical fitness, and obese but fit individuals can live just as long as their fit counterparts with normal BMI.

Some experts have proposed countering the weaknesses of BMI by substituting other measures, such as waist circumference or waist-to-hip ratio. These methods show some promise, but BMI remains the most commonly used measure in clinical practice. Ultimately though, it is important to realize that a number on the scale is just one component of physical fitness.

Throughout this chapter, I have tried to emphasize that exercise is not a great weight loss solution. Plenty of people start increasing their physical activity, only to be discouraged and stop when they fail in their weight loss goals. But as the data on exercise clearly show, physical activity transcends weight loss, providing us with longer, healthier lives regardless of our weight.

How can we use all this information to become healthier people? Unless we are the rare person doing ten times the recommended amount of exercise, the answer is simple: we should all work harder to increase our level of physical activity. These changes can be small, like parking far away from the entrance when we go to the store or committing to taking the stairs instead of the elevator. They can also be much bigger, like training for a big race or taking up a new sport. Regardless, the secret to a healthier life is clear – you just have to keep moving.

CHAPTER 4: SLEEP

WHY HOSPITAL DOCTORS LOVE MELATONIN

It is no secret that patients sleep poorly in the hospital. But sometimes, it seems like hospital staff are actively working to keep their patients awake. Instead of being comfortable at home, patients are tasked with trying to sleep in an uncomfortable hospital bed while hooked up to IVs and beeping monitors. Patients who manage to ignore these distractions are frequently woken up by nurses checking vital signs. If they are able to drift back off, overhead code announcements and frequent footsteps in the hallway help ensure they cannot stay asleep for long. As a result, patients end up sleeping considerably less in the hospital than they do at home. One study of hospitalized patients reported that, on average, patients only slept 5.5 hours a night. Meanwhile, experts from the American Academy of Sleep Medicine and the Sleep Research Society both recommend that adults sleep at least seven hours a night. In other words, we might actually be hurting our patients by depriving them of sleep while they should be recovering.

Lack of sleep has been the subject of many morning conversations I have had with hospitalized patients who are understandably upset at being unable to rest at night. Unfortunately, there is little that we as healthcare providers can do to help. Those IVs, while annoying, are delivering important drugs. The monitors help us make sure all our patients are stable. And the hospital is a 24/7 workplace, meaning there is always a chance that some external commotion may disturb the peace and wake people up.

These excuses often mean little to patients, who want to know what specifically can be done to make their next night in the hospital more restful. As a result, many doctors offer a low dose of melatonin to hospitalized patients. Melatonin is a hormone that helps regulate the sleep-wake cycle, and it has been used for years in pill form as a supplement to promote improved sleep. That being said, melatonin cannot magically make the discomfort of an IV or the beeping of a monitor disappear, meaning that 24 hours later, patient and doctor often find themselves once again locked in a dispute over nighttime distractions. Some doctors, essentially for lack of a better solution, will offer to increase the dose of melatonin.

Melatonin has now provided the doctor with two days of excuses for their patients' poor sleep in the hospital. In a busy doctor's day, with life and death often on the line, it is easy to brush patient concerns about sleep away and try to solve the problem with a simple promise of melatonin. But is the melatonin actually providing any benefit to the patient?

For as much as doctors are frequently skeptical of supplements, melatonin is a supplement that certainly works.

But, contrary to how some doctors make it sound to their sleepy patients, it is hardly a miracle cure for insomnia. Researchers examined various studies investigating melatonin's effects on sleep. They found that, on average, melatonin helped people fall asleep seven minutes faster and ultimately sleep eight minutes longer than a placebo. But while a scientific study might conclude that this result is statistically significant, it is easy to argue that a mere eight extra minutes of sleep is hardly worth taking the pill.

Sure, there are other, much stronger, sleeping pills. But the beauty of melatonin is that, unlike stronger sleep aids, it is not habit forming and has relatively limited side effects. A safe, easy-to-quit sleep aid makes sense in the hospital, where vulnerable patients are frequently already taking a wide variety of potentially interacting medications. But even outside the hospital, many doctors are hesitant to prescribe anything more than melatonin for trouble with sleep. I have seen patients who have become so dependent on sleep medications that they essentially cannot sleep without them. I have also witnessed patients try prescription-strength sleeping medications just once and claim the side effects made them never want to see a sleeping pill again. There are lots of people who struggle with sleep, but few people who want to be beholden to a drug in order to get that sleep.

The Centers for Disease Control (CDC) report that 35% of Americans sleep less than seven hours a night on average, failing to meet recommendations for the minimum amount of sleep. The nation's sleeplessness might be worsening over time, as evidence shows more Americans sleep less than six hours a night than they did a generation ago. There are good reasons to explain our lack of sleep. Unlike most of human history, we are now inundated with electric light, giving us the option to work or play during dark hours when our ancestors' activities would have been limited. We also lead busy, stressful lives, often preventing us from getting into bed in the first place or leaving our brain active once we get there.

Research has shown that there are some people who are genetically predisposed to function better on limited sleep. For the vast majority of us, however, lack of sleep does have consequences. As expected, people tend to do worse on cognitive tasks when sleep deprived. Pretty much everyone has felt the mental drain from a poor night of sleep every once in a while. But we do not even necessarily need to feel tired to suffer the effects of limited sleep. In one study, researchers surveyed subjects on their typical sleep habits and asked whether or not they had been in a car accident during the previous year. Individuals reporting six hours of sleep a night were 33% more likely to have been in an accident than people who slept seven or eight hours a night. The increased risk of a car accident was seen across all sleep-deprived individuals, not just in people who reported excessive sleepiness.

Lack of sleep can even make you more susceptible to sickness. When a different set of researchers exposed volunteers to a common cold virus, individuals reporting less than seven hours of sleep were three times as likely to get sick than those sleeping eight or more hours a night. A separate study showed individuals sleeping less than six hours a night had a 20% higher risk of a heart attack than their counterparts who slept between six and nine hours a night.

Even without being experts on the risks associated with lack of sleep, many people have a simple solution to daytime sleepiness – a nap. Researchers have found benefits of naps, and generally suggest naps should last about twenty minutes. These short naps can lead to decreased sleepiness and improved cognitive function after reawakening. However, researchers tend to notice what they call sleep inertia, defined as a period of drowsiness after waking up, with longer naps. Naps leading to sleep inertia, generally 30 minutes or longer, may therefore be less useful than shorter naps. Of course, forcing a strict limit on a nap is not necessarily easy. Maybe that is why Americans report that their naps are a full hour long, on average. Regardless, naps are not necessarily a cure for lack of sleep at night. Even after daytime naps, study subjects who had been chronically sleep restricted still showed decreased cognitive function and mood. In the same study, mankind's other technique to solve sleepiness, caffeine, also failed to restore subjects to baseline.

Naps can be useful, but the sleep research cautions against more exotic sleeping strategies. Breaking up sleep into anything more than a main period of sleep and a nap is called polyphasic sleeping. Polyphasic sleeping is essentially extreme napping, often at the expense of the total number of hours slept. Online, it is not hard to find claims that famous luminaries were able to perform at the top of their fields with limited sleep due to polyphasic sleeping. Famed inventor Thomas Edison purported to only sleep four or five hours each night. Noted architect Buckminster Fuller claimed to work with only four half-hour naps a day, each nap spaced out every six hours. But when sleep scientists reviewed studies on polyphasic sleeping strategies, they found that the vast majority of the evidence pointed toward these strategies being ineffective, with negative effects on cognitive function.

So, sleep is important, and people are not getting enough of it. But what are the options for people who have trouble sleeping? The issue with answering this question is that sleeping troubles are not as easy to solve as problems with diet or exercise. A poor diet can be fixed with healthier eating.

Inactivity can be solved by getting off the couch. But you cannot just tell someone to sleep more. There is an incredibly long list of causes for poor sleep, from mental blocks on sleep like stress and anxiety to underlying medical causes like sleep apnea and chronic pain. Different causes of poor sleep have different solutions. The continuous positive airway pressure (CPAP) machine a doctor might prescribe for the patient with sleep apnea certainly is not the solution for the patient struggling with anxiety.

Since sleep is such a complex issue, people struggling with chronic sleep issues may benefit from talking over their symptoms and concerns with a doctor. There is even a medical specialty, sleep medicine, dedicated to addressing patients' sleep-related concerns. Sleep medicine doctors might not be as well known to the public as cardiologists or neurologists, but their existence shows that sleep disorders alone can form the basis of an entire medical specialty.

Thankfully, there are strategies that in theory can help us improve both the quantity and the quality of our sleep. Sleep researchers group these solutions under the concept of sleep hygiene. Sleep hygiene focuses on setting ourselves up for a good night of sleep by doing things like going to bed at a consistent time, limiting bright lights late at night, and avoiding caffeine before bed. Sleep hygiene tips make a lot of sense, but they can also sound a little bit like sleep researchers scolding us for living our lives: Drink less coffee! Turn off the TV! Don't stay up late on the weekends! Do these tips actually hold up when studied?

Here is where the evidence gets a little confusing. In small studies looking at individual components of sleep hygiene, the suggestions seem to help. For example, one of the most common sleep hygiene tips is to perform physical activity during the day. The logic is simple. Physical activity makes us tired, and tired people sleep well at night. And when test subjects were randomized to either complete a triweekly exercise program or serve as inactive controls, individuals who exercised reported better sleep.

However, having good sleep hygiene does not necessarily equal a better night of sleep. A separate study examined nursing home residents given a multicomponent sleep hygiene regimen. They increased their physical activity, had at least 30 minutes of sunlight exposure, reduced their time awake in bed during the day, and followed a strict bedtime routine. While individuals practicing sleep hygiene took less daytime naps and were more alert during the day, researchers found no significant difference in total nighttime sleep between the sleep hygiene practitioners and a control group.

One negative study does not disprove the concept of sleep hygiene. Still, some sleep researchers have noticed large discrepancies between sleep hygiene recommendations and the actual evidence from studies. One example is daytime napping. The general sleep hygiene recommendation is to avoid daytime naps. On the surface, the logic here makes perfect sense. A little rest during the day might hurt our ability to fall asleep at night. However, the evidence fails to back this claim up, as most research demonstrates that naps actually have little impact on nighttime sleep. Similarly, sleep hygiene emphasizes the need to maintain a consistent sleep schedule. Again, this makes sense in theory. But studies requiring participants to maintain a consistent sleep schedule have not always found increases in total sleep.

Obtaining high-quality evidence on sleep hygiene recommendations can be extraordinarily difficult, as many sleep studies have to be done in a controlled environment. A study that regulated participants' sleep schedule used college students as subjects, and required them to sleep for 38 consecutive nights in a research laboratory. This study design practically begs us to question if the effects on sleep seen during the study were due to the sleep schedule, or instead from the new, uninviting sleep environment.

Outside of the laboratory, turning sleep hygiene recommendations into sleep improvements can be even more difficult. When doctors offer sleep hygiene tips, we run the risk of believing that educating our patients on sleep hygiene fundamentals will automatically translate to patients making changes. Think back to the study on nursing home residents. In that study, the large amount of assistance nursing home residents receive on a daily basis, coupled with the controlled nature of a scientific experiment, meant that sleep hygiene techniques could actually be implemented. In contrast, if I tell a patient struggling with insomnia to increase their physical activity and keep a consistent sleep schedule, I have no way of knowing if they will follow my advice.

As such, sleep hygiene recommendations have two strikes against them. First, while some of the tips do hold up to scientific scrutiny, others are hardly settled science. And second, it is unclear if teaching individuals about sleep hygiene actually makes a difference in how they sleep. I like to view sleep hygiene recommendations as a starting point for patients who suffer from chronic insomnia. After all, it is unlikely that asking my patients to try an afternoon walk or to limit nighttime light exposure will do any harm. One of the biggest strengths of sleep hygiene recommendations is that they are meant to be easy adjustments with no obvious downsides or significant side effects. But I think it is also important to be honest with patients and tell them these changes do not work for everyone.

That being said, there have been some clear successes in the sleep medicine community. Temperature changes of as little as one degree Fahrenheit have been shown to have dramatic effects on sleep quality, suggesting that the body is exquisitely sensitive to temperature at night. Many experts claim that a bedroom should be kept around 65 degrees, much cooler than common daytime room temperatures, in order to facilitate sleep. As such, some insomniacs might reap big improvements from subtle changes to their nighttime temperature settings.

People who are willing to put a little more effort into improving their sleep may also benefit from a specific therapy designed to tackle the root causes of their sleeplessness. This therapy, called Cognitive Behavioral Therapy for Insomnia (CBT-I), has been shown to be efficacious in improving sleep. In one study, subjects randomly assigned to CBT-I slept 40 more minutes on average than subjects assigned to receive sleep hygiene education. In the sleep medicine literature, where we are expected to be thrilled about eight minutes of extra sleep with melatonin, 40 extra minutes of sleep is a huge deal.

Unfortunately, stigmas around therapy might dissuade many people from trying CBT-I. There is also a concern that because CBT-I is by definition a short-term intervention, chronic insomniacs might return to their old, poor sleeping patterns after the program concludes. Still, the fact that a few sessions of targeted therapy can lead to a sizable increase in total sleep suggests that we can be doing a lot more to help our insomniacs get some rest. The effectiveness of therapy at helping improve sleep also demonstrates just how powerful the mind can be in determining whether our body gets to bed. Sleep hygiene recommendations, like refraining from evening caffeine or avoiding bright lights before bed, generally rest on the concept of preparing our body for sleep. But the effectiveness of CBT-I demonstrates that preparing our mind to sleep might be even more effective. Perhaps that is why weighted blankets have been found to be effective in improving sleep for people who suffer from depression and anxiety. Research also shows that mindfulness and meditation may play a role in improving sleep.

As a doctor, I think therapy can be enormously helpful. I also think there are some people who would rather never sleep again than have to chat with a therapist. That is not necessarily a bad thing. For every person who needs to work on their mind-body connection to have better sleep, there is another person who probably just needs to turn off their phone and get their butt in bed a bit earlier. Ultimately, the best recommendation for improved sleep is an individual approach. In the chapters on diet and exercise, we learned that pretty much any diet and pretty much any form of physical activity can be beneficial. Studies examining sleep, on the other hand, show that many interventions have limited effects on average. There is no one-size-fits-all solution to a good night's sleep.

Still, the lack of a simple solution does not mean we should all resign ourselves to poor sleep. Just because something has limited effects on average does not mean it cannot work well for certain individuals. While melatonin only leads to eight more minutes of sleep on average, it personally does wonders for me. Studies may show sleep hygiene to have modest effects, but any one person still might notice a huge improvement from subtle changes in sleep habits. Experimenting with things like room temperature, weighted blankets, and maybe even therapy can all be extraordinarily helpful in improving sleep. There can be a better night's sleep out there for everyone. We just have to figure out what works for us.

CHAPTER 5: PAIN

WHY A TOOTHPICK MIGHT HELP AN ACHING BACK

Being in pain is never fun. But at least we can take solace in the fact that pain is incredibly common. The CDC estimates that in a given three-month period, more than half of Americans will report some sort of pain. Back pain is the most common complaint, but any body part can hurt, from a throbbing headache all the way down to a jammed toe. The causes of some pain, like a sprained ankle from tripping on stairs or an aching elbow after a game of tennis, can be obvious. But other pains, often more chronic or hard to describe, can be quite mysterious. Both to figure out what exactly is causing their pain, as well as for advice on how to get rid of it, people naturally turn to their doctors for advice.

These visits, for us doctors, can range from simple to extraordinarily complex. It is not hard to figure out the cause of someone's back pain if they reported lifting heavy boxes two days ago, then felt the pain the next morning. However, a patient's chronic back pain can be from a dizzying array of causes. Sure, this sort of back pain can be from simple overuse or normal aging. But anything and everything from disseminated tuberculosis to metastatic cancer could also theoretically be the cause.

Patients who only want reassurance that their pain is not coming from some insidious source are generally pretty easy to treat. Years of medical training, plus a few simple tests, can often help their doctors rule out the scariest diagnoses. Unfortunately, when people start asking for how best to treat their pain, doctors are often in a bind.

Modern medicine has made some illnesses extremely easy to treat. Give me a patient with diabetes, and I can use medications to control their blood sugars. Give a surgeon an inflamed appendix, and they can remove it with a minimally invasive surgery. But for how common pain is, doctors still are not that great at treating it.

The perfect example might be acetaminophen (often branded as Tylenol), one of the oldest and most commonly used pain medications. Picture the classic pain scale that doctors use, where patients are asked to rate their pain from zero to ten. Ideally, an effective pain medication would be able to lower pain by a large amount, say from a seven to a three. Optimists might even argue that modern medicine should be able to eliminate unwanted pain entirely. But when scientists examined how effective acetaminophen was for reducing pain from knee or hip arthritis, they found that patients' pain ratings only dropped by 0.3 points on average.

"Gee, thanks, doc." I can imagine my patients saying sarcastically. A drop of 0.3 points out of 10 would seem for most of us to be little more than a rounding error. Somehow, acetaminophen is even less effective for some other conditions. For acute low back pain, the same researchers could not clearly say that acetaminophen worked at all.

Other common pain relievers tend to fall into a category called non-steroidal anti-inflammatory medications (NSAIDs). These drugs include medicine cabinet staples like ibuprofen, aspirin, and naproxen. Unfortunately, their efficacy also seems to be less than thrilling. One study examined whether subjects with headaches still had pain two hours after taking ibuprofen. Only 23% of people who took ibuprofen reported resolution of their headaches. That sounds disappointing enough, but consider that 16% of people in a separate placebo group also reported that their headache went away. Accounting for the placebo, ibuprofen only seemed to help 7% of the test subjects. Better than nothing, but hardly a miracle drug.

All the drugs we have discussed so far are available over the counter, meaning without a prescription from a doctor. And because they are limited in their effectiveness, it is no wonder that many patients come to their doctors looking for something stronger. For many patients, this means opioids.

Even acknowledging all their controversy, opioids remain extraordinarily effective against pain. In one study, morphine and fentanyl, two common opioids, took only 15 minutes to lower average pain scores from 6.8 out of 10 to just 1.4 out of 10. In that study, more than 80% of patients reported satisfaction with the pain control the opioid medications provided.

The astounding efficacy of opioids is not new knowledge. Opium itself is naturally produced by the *Papaver somniferum* poppy plant, and references to its medicinal uses date back to ancient Mesopotamian cultures, where it was called 'the joy plant.' In 1844, Irish physician Francis Rynd created the first hollow needle, which was specifically designed to allow him to administer an opioid more directly. Per Rynd's report, his patient's pain disappeared in less than a minute.

Of course, the dangers of opioids are not new either. Over 100 years ago, the Harrison Anti-Narcotic Act was enacted to better regulate opioid use, setting strict rules for opioid prescriptions. In the 1980s and 1990s, however, sentiment shifted, and it was thought that the development of longer-acting opioid formulations would temper the risk of addiction. Unfortunately, this was not the case, and death rates from prescription opioids increased nearly 400% between 1999 and 2009.

In recent years, opioid prescriptions have been falling, although the opioid epidemic rages on. The CDC guidelines on prescribing opioids note that over 100 million opioid prescriptions are still dispensed annually, and that opioids remain the most commonly misused prescription drug, with almost ten million Americans reporting opioid misuse.

The CDC guidelines add that only 11% of people misusing opioids state they do so to "feel good or get high." In contrast, the vast majority of people misusing opioids report doing so to relieve pain. The goal of pain management, not a high, is the reason why the CDC uses the term misuse, not abuse, to describe these actions. So, the real question is not "why do people abuse opioids?" Instead, we should ask, "why are people taking these medicines and still in such pain?" Interestingly, while opioids remain effective at treating acute pain, more and more evidence has emerged that opioids might actually be bad for chronic pain. The CDC notes that chronic opioid use is actually associated with worse long-term outcomes for common conditions like arthritis, low back pain, and headache.

One fascinating theory for the worsening outcomes associated with chronic opioid use is something called opioid-induced hyperalgesia. Put more simply, the idea is that opioids rewire our brain chemistry, making us more susceptible to painful stimuli. This concept makes a lot of sense. Pain is our body's way of telling us that something is wrong. Opioids work by blocking that messaging system. In response, our body has to make the pain signals feel stronger, which can lead to increased chronic pain.

It is a little disconcerting to think about the fact that our bodies are forcing us to feel pain, but we must also consider that the inability to feel pain is dangerous too. Some people are born with a condition called congenital analgesia, which means they lack any ability to sense pain. At first, this sounds like a superpower. But pain, however uncomfortable, gives us an important message that something is wrong. Many reports of congenital analgesia in the scientific literature involve the patient presenting with some terribly advanced condition, like a serious bone infection, that they were unaware of due to their inability to feel pain.

The takeaway here is that even if there were some magic pill to relieve all pain, doctors could not prescribe it without consequences. And as we have discussed, the medications that we do have at our disposal are far from magic cures. Admittedly, we have only covered a few common types of pain medication. There are other pain pills too, including medications like cyclobenzaprine, baclofen, and tizanidine, which are frequently grouped into a class called muscle relaxers. Some antidepressant drugs are frequently used to control pain as well. But as you might guess, these medications are not without their side effects, and might be more widely known if they were more effective.

Clearly, there is a market for better products to control pain. Perhaps that is why some people turn to street drugs for pain management. Somewhat ironically, the medical field itself has embraced some of these treatments as well. Ketamine used to be best known as a hallucinogen that could give people an illicit trip, but is now being evaluated as a solution for chronic pain. Medical marijuana's availability has exploded in recent years, and one of its most notable uses is for pain management.

Of course, these newer treatments are not the only options that people are turning to for their pain. There are plenty of tried and true alternatives as well. Acupuncture, where needles are placed into the skin to control pain, has been used for thousands of years. While such a procedure might invoke skepticism, multiple studies have found it to be effective in decreasing subjective pain ratings. Still, there remains a great deal of controversy over whether acupuncture needles are actually doing something. One study compared real acupuncture with simulated acupuncture, where trained acupuncturists used toothpick pricks to make subjects think they were getting the real thing. The result? Both the toothpick acupuncture and the real acupuncture led to similar decreases in pain.

There are two ways to interpret this study. The first is that whatever pain-fighting property acupuncture offers seems to be accomplished much more simply with a toothpick. Perhaps there is some truth to this interpretation, and a small amount of temporary pain, whether through acupuncture needles or a toothpick, can decrease chronic pain. In a way, this is strikingly similar to how short-term pain relief with opioids can actually worsen pain over the long term.

The second interpretation is that simply receiving a treatment, even if it is just a toothpick prick to the back, can make a meaningful difference in people's perception of pain. I think us doctors need to take the second interpretation much more seriously. I am sure that many of my colleagues scoff at patients who report going to spiritual or energy-based healers because these treatments fail to fit in with evidence-based Western medicine. But people return to these practices over and over again, probably because something about the care they receive there is making them feel better.

When patients go to their doctor complaining of pain, they are looking for us to do something about it. But as we have learned, a lot of our medications to address pain are far from perfect. At the same time, pain will frequently resolve on its own with rest and time, meaning that doctors who suggest extremely conservative treatment approaches to pain are often doing the right thing. Of course, their patients might be unhappy with such a passive approach. This discrepancy between patient expectations and physician pain management choices can lead to frustration from both sides.

One of the biggest disconnects between patients and doctors when it comes to pain management relates to imaging tests, like X-rays and magnetic resonance imaging (MRI). Patients tend to expect this sort of evaluation when they come to their doctor complaining of pain. And yet, there is ample evidence that for some specific complaints, this sort of imaging does not improve pain outcomes at all. Think of it like this. A lot of pain comes from muscular and skeletal causes, like torn ligaments resulting in a sprain, worn down cartilage between bones causing arthritis, and overstretched tendons with small tears. X-rays can see bony changes, and MRI can see more of the other tissues, but the knowledge of what specifically is causing the pain does not always make treatment more successful.

In fact, it can be hard to tell if abnormalities seen on

these imaging studies are actually what is causing the pain in the first place. Tears to the knee menisci, which are small pieces of cartilage that help cushion the knee, are a common reason for knee pain. And yet, they can also be found incidentally on an MRI as well, implying that they do not always cause pain when present. So, if I order an MRI on a patient complaining of knee pain, I might find an incidental meniscus tear that the patient will then want surgically fixed, even if it is not clear that the tear is what is causing the patient's pain. Interestingly, even among patients who do undergo surgery to repair meniscus tears, there is not great evidence that surgery offers any better long-term pain relief than physical therapy alone.

There is some personal bias here, but I think that physical therapy is a nice compromise between patients wanting something active to do for their pain and doctors tending to treat injuries conservatively. I send a lot of patients to physical therapy for their pain, and there is good evidence that physical activity is an effective way to make people in pain feel better, often requiring less healthcare dollars than more intensive interventions.

Of course, there are a lot of people who lack the time or the money to go to physical therapy appointments. Other patients will try physical therapy and not see much benefit. Luckily, patients who fail to benefit from one type of therapy can feel much better with other options. Guidelines published by the American College of Physicians for the treatment of low back pain recommend a wide variety of conservative options. Some of these options we have already discussed, like NSAIDs and acupuncture. Again, these are not miracle cures by any stretch of the imagination. But they can certainly help. Other guideline recommendations include various forms of physical therapy, massage, mindfulness-based meditation, tai chi, yoga, progressive relaxation, and cognitive behavioral therapy.

Skeptics might note that I already addressed the controversy behind acupuncture's effectiveness, and should rightfully question how mental therapies such as meditation adequately address physical causes of pain. If this is a book about evidence-based medicine, why would I mention treatments with such questionable evidence?

I'll be honest, when I recently broke a toe, I did not start meditating or poking myself with toothpicks to simulate acupuncture. Instead, I grabbed some ibuprofen and gradually returned to my regular level of activity. But I also think it is important for both patients and doctors to understand that pain involves neural pathways, and as such is just as much a mental phenomenon as it is a physical one. Emergency room doctors are taught to evaluate for 'distracting injuries', or injuries causing patients to ignore other sources of pain. Think of a patient being in so much pain from one broken bone that they fail to notice a second, smaller, fracture. The idea here is that our body is able to ignore an injury that would normally cause us a great deal of pain, but only when distracted by something even worse.

Obviously, the solution to everyday aches and pains is not to give ourselves a more serious injury, but the example shows that our response to pain involves complex physical, neurological, and psychological pathways. Many of the guideline recommended options focus on treatments that take advantage of this interplay. So yes, acupuncture and meditation may not directly fix the underlying causes of chronic pain, but if they make my patients feel better, I won't complain.

Just because doctors do not have a magic solution for pain does not mean that we are useless to our patients when something is hurting. But it is probably a good idea to temper expectations. Doctors are pretty good at differentiating between pain that is a sign of something dangerous and pain that is relatively benign. However, we are less good at making that relatively benign pain go away completely. While our patients can become understandably frustrated when pain persists, partnering with a doctor to help ensure treatments are safe and sensible can go a long way.

Pain is common, and our treatments are far from perfect. But there is a large and growing array of options we have for pain management. A good doctor should know when just giving an injury time to heal is the best strategy, but should also have plenty of other options to offer as backup.

CHAPTER 6: VITAMINS AND SUPPLEMENTS

WHY VITAMIN A MAY HAVE KILLED AN ANTARCTIC EXPLORER

In 1911, explorers Douglas Mawson, Belgrave Ninnis, and Xavier Mertz set out to explore a previously unmapped section of the Antarctic. Tragically, it proved to be an ill-fated expedition. Ninnis fell into a crevasse along with most of the trio's supplies, leading to his death and forcing Mawson and Mertz to continue with little food. Almost two months later, an emaciated Mawson was the only one to reach the end of the expedition, with Mertz having died after suffering weeks of scanty rations. What killed Mertz? As Mawson was the only one to witness his decline and death, there is some controversy on the topic. Mertz may have simply died secondary to starvation and constant exposure to the frigid Antarctic. But some researchers have latched onto a second theory, that Mertz died from an overdose of vitamin A.

How could a starving explorer overdose on a vitamin? A common yet mistaken belief is that we should all be trying to ingest as many vitamins as possible. Plenty of organic food fans lambast the chemicals in our processed diets, saying we should instead focus on foods filled with natural vitamins. This sort of argument is pervasive in the world of healthy eating, and it does make some sense. Yet, vitamins are chemicals too, just like anything and everything that we eat. The word vitamin itself is short for 'vital amines', meaning amines (a type of chemical) that early researchers thought were important to vital processes. A vital amine is something you certainly want to have in your diet. But as Mertz learned the hard way, having too much of a vitamin is not necessarily a good thing.

The theory of Mertz dying from an overdose of vitamin A goes like this. While Antarctic explorers brought food rations with them for their expeditions, Inuit tribes had been living in similarly harsh conditions in the Arctic for centuries. Inuit tribes survived on a largely meat-based diet, hunting Arctic creatures like polar bear and seal. But the Inuit learned to avoid eating polar bear and seal liver, as it could cause a violent sickness. European explorers, lacking this knowledge, had multiple expeditions suffer severe disease after members ate polar bear liver. Much later, researchers learned that liver meat in general is a high source of vitamin A, and that polar bear and seal liver contained so much vitamin A that it was toxic. Mawson and Mertz, stranded with limited supplies in the Antarctic, adopted a meat-heavy diet much like the Inuit on the other side of the world. In their desperation for any source of food, they were forced to kill and eat their dogs, which they ate, liver and all. For

Mertz, who rarely ate any meat in his regular diet, the vitamin A dose may have simply been too much.

Modern Americans have the luxury of a little more variety in our diet. Unlike our ancestors or people in famine-stricken areas of the world, we do not have to worry about nasty diseases associated with vitamin deficiencies like beriberi, pellagra, or scurvy. And while it lacks a fancy name, vitamin A deficiency is not a pleasant thing. In addition to weakening the immune system, vitamin A deficiency is most famously associated with impaired vision. The idea of treating vision impairments with vitamin A goes all the way back to Ancient Egypt, where the cure for night blindness was known to be, as you might now guess, liver. Vitamin A supplementation is still used in developing nations to prevent deficiencies that can lead to infant mortality. Trials have shown that these supplements can literally be life-saving.

But even in wealthy nations, where vitamin A deficiency is rare, many people obsess over eating enough vitamins. Vitamin A supplements are available in almost every pharmacy, and Vitamin A is generally included in multivitamin supplements as well. About 30% of Americans are estimated to take a supplement that includes vitamin A. The logic here is that if some vitamin A is necessary, more should be better. Some people go further, arguing that extra vitamins, through their antioxidant power, should be able to tame aging and reduce the risk of cancer. Is there any truth here?

Well, one study showed that a multivitamin supplement including vitamins A, C, and E, in addition to zinc, reduced the risk of developing macular degeneration, a progressive vision impairment. Of course, a different formulation of the supplement, without any vitamin A, reduced the risk just as much. Vitamin A was removed from the formula because two other studies showed an association between vitamin A supplementation and an increased risk of lung cancer. That association is scary, but also shows up repeatedly. Even in the study on macular degeneration, people taking the supplement with vitamin A were more likely to develop lung cancer. There is also a concerning association between high levels of vitamin A and an increased risk of osteoporosis and fracture.

The example of vitamin A demonstrates that while vitamins are certainly necessary to avoid disease, more is not necessarily better. People tend to pop vitamin supplements like they are no big deal, but vitamins, just like prescription medications, are chemicals with a long list of potential side effects. Thankfully, not every vitamin has the side effect profile of vitamin A. Unlike fat-soluble vitamin A, which can build up in body tissues chronically, the B vitamins are water-soluble. As such, excess B vitamins are more easily excreted in urine.

Just like with vitamin A, you definitely want to have enough B vitamins in your diet. Deficiencies in B vitamins are linked to a whole host of neurological disorders, cognitive disorders, a weakened immune system, and even cardiovascular complications. While wealthy nations tend to have easy access to calories, studies still show that plenty of Americans have B vitamin deficiencies. Does that mean we should all be taking B vitamin supplements? One study showed that higher levels of Vitamin B2, also known as riboflavin, is associated with lower rates of lung cancer. Increased levels of Vitamin B6, also known as pyridoxine, have been linked to lower risks of prostate cancer. However, there is a big difference between studies showing these general associations and studies showing a clear benefit from B vitamin supplementation. Unfortunately, an analysis of 18 different studies all looking at B vitamin supplementation and cancer risk found that adding a B vitamin supplement did not affect cancer incidence, death due to cancer, or overall mortality.

Vitamin C has perhaps the most famous backstory of any vitamin, as many people know the link between sailors deprived of vitamin C on long voyages and the development of scurvy. Well before the discovery of vitamin C, Captain James Cook tried and failed to prevent scurvy with treatments like sweet wort and spruce beer. After the actual chemical compound had been discovered and shown to cure scurvy, Nobel-winning chemist Linus Pauling argued that high doses of vitamin C could be used to prevent infections such as the common cold. Winning a Nobel Prize on one subject, however, does not mean that every theory you have is correct. Other scientists have repeatedly questioned the actual efficacy of vitamin C in preventing colds. Still, the public perception of Vitamin C as a miracle drug stuck. Vitamin C consumption doubled in two years after Linus Pauling started speaking in favor if its use, and its miraculous (though unproven) benefits were extended to other diseases as well. Today, vitamin C is claimed to help treat or prevent everything from preeclampsia to COVID-19, without substantial direct evidence to back up these claims. On the other hand, vitamin C has been proven to have no effect on the risk of stroke, no effect on cancer prevention, and no effect on cardiovascular disease.

Since so many people take vitamin C supplements when they have a cold, and many people swear by it as a common cold treatment, I want to dive deeper into the data on vitamin C and colds. An analysis of 29 placebo-controlled studies on vitamin C supplementation, involving over 11,000 subjects, showed that vitamin C supplementation was associated with a 5% decreased risk of developing a cold. A 5% decrease is technically a positive result, but it is hardly a game-changing strategy for cold prevention. Importantly, some of those studies were done on special groups like marathon runners and Canadian troops stationed in subarctic conditions. These studies might not be applicable to the overall population. After removing these groups from the analysis, there was no statistically significant difference in the risk of people developing colds based on whether or not they were taking a vitamin C supplement. Of course, vitamin C proponents also argue that vitamin C can shorten the length of a cold as well. An analysis of 31 studies on vitamin C supplements and the length of cold symptoms found that, on average, there was a minor reduction in the length of cold symptoms with vitamin C supplementation. The effect was significant, if rather modest, with adults seeing an 8% reduction in length of cold symptoms and children having a 14% reduction. Doctors who haughtily tell their patients that vitamin C supplements are completely useless are probably overstating their case, but patients who swear by vitamin C as a common cold cure are similarly overconfident.

Still, even something as benign as vitamin C can have its side effects. One study found an association between vitamin C supplementation and men developing kidney stones. A separate case report describes a young man developing ultimately fatal cardiomyopathy after ingesting large doses of vitamin C. These findings complicate the concept of giving large doses of vitamin C in the hope of making cold symptoms go away a few hours earlier.

Vitamin D supplements are also discussed as a possible cold-busting solution. One study found higher levels of vitamin D in the blood were associated with a decreased risk of respiratory infections. However, these associations do not mean the vitamin D is causing a stronger immune response. The same result would hold true if people who were deficient in vitamin D were simply less healthy in general, and therefore more likely to fall prey to a respiratory infection. In fact, an explanation like this one makes more sense than vitamin D itself being the underlying cause. After all, two separate high quality randomized-controlled trials both showed that supplementing vitamin D failed to reduce the risk of upper respiratory infections.

Unlike the other vitamins, very few foods are good sources of vitamin D. Instead, most of our vitamin D production is through exposure to sunlight. But the strength of the sunlight also seems to matter, meaning that a sunny day during summer in the tropics is likely to lead to a whole lot more vitamin D production than a sunny day during winter in Canada. As a lot of the world's population lives in areas with cold winters, vitamin D deficiency is common throughout the world, with an estimated 1 billion people having low vitamin D levels. Although it is common, vitamin D deficiency is associated with some scary stuff. An increased risk of cancer, an increased chance of developing diabetes, and an increased risk of inflammatory bowel disease are just some of associations connected to low levels of vitamin D. But again, noticing these associations is not the same as believing that low vitamin D causes these diseases. If there were a direct link of causation between low vitamin D and these disease states, we would expect vitamin D supplementation to lower the risk of developing these diseases. Unfortunately, vitamin D supplementation has not been convincingly shown to decrease the risk of cancer, diabetes, or a whole host of other disease states associated with low vitamin D.

Still, these findings do not mean that vitamin D supplementation is useless. After all, vitamin D plays an important role in healthy bone maintenance, and many people have vitamin D deficiencies. Some studies have shown a reduction in mortality with vitamin D supplementation, especially in groups like the elderly that are frequently deficient in vitamin D. There is definitely some controversy here, and guideline groups including the United States Preventive Service Task Force do not even recommend general screening of patients for vitamin D deficiencies. And there certainly is no guideline recommending that every man, woman, and child start supplementing with vitamin D. Yet, when doctors do find vitamin D deficiencies (often by testing in violation of the above guideline), they are generally encouraged to treat them. After all, there is some evidence that vitamin D supplementation might reduce falls and the risk of fractures in older adults, especially in patients who are vitamin D deficient. But picking up on low vitamin D levels can be difficult, as symptoms can be as vague as low back pain or muscle aches.

The guidelines are confusing, both for patients and doctors. I already noted that there is evidence arguing vitamin D supplementation is unlikely to reduce the rates of upper respiratory infections. But there is also evidence that for individuals with very low levels of vitamin D, supplementation actually could help decrease the risk of the common cold. And without regular screening for vitamin D deficiency, doctors would have no way to determine who might benefit from extra vitamin D. As more studies are done, we may see both guidelines and clinical practice change. For now, I do not tell all my patients to start taking vitamin D, but I also certainly would not force committed patients to stop taking a reasonable dose as a supplement.

On the other hand, I would be much more skeptical of a patient's vitamin E supplement. Vitamin E is known as an antioxidant that can help rid the body of free radicals. Since free radicals are thought to contribute to cancer, one could arrive at the conclusion that vitamin E supplementation could be a powerful anticancer tool used to extend lives. However, the evidence does not back up this claim. Not only do studies examining vitamin E supplementation fail to show an increase in lifespan, but high dose vitamin E supplementation may actually increase the risk of dying.

Despite the mixed data, tens of millions of Americans still spend money on vitamins and supplements each year. It has been estimated that total U.S. sales of supplements are around $28 billion. That represents as much money as the entire yearly economy of Honduras, a country of over 10 million people. Sure, some individual studies have found a benefit here or there. But as a whole, benefits of vitamin supplements are small or nonexistent at best. An editorial in The Annals of Internal Medicine, a prestigious medical journal, sums up some experts' viewpoints on supplements with its title alone: "Enough is enough: stop wasting money on vitamin and mineral supplements." Personally, I would argue that such a viewpoint is somewhat of an oversimplification. We have already discussed small but positive effects of vitamin C supplements on shortening cold symptoms as well as a multivitamin supplement that decreased the risk of macular degeneration. Are these incremental, frequently controversial benefits worth $28 billion a year? That, I will admit, is a different question altogether.

The one vitamin that doctors do seem to agree on is also the big vitamin we have yet to discuss – vitamin K. Unlike the other vitamins, however, vitamin K supplements are largely meant for newborns. Vitamin K plays an important role in our blood, helping it to clot when necessary. Newborns, however, are frequently deficient in vitamin K, putting them at risk for potentially life-threatening bleeding. A vitamin K injection given just after birth decreases the risk of these bleeds, helping keep the baby safe. Ironically, the vitamin that doctors feel has the best evidence is also the one that we have the most trouble convincing patients to allow us to administer. A growing number of parents have been refusing the vitamin K injection, arguing that is unnecessary and unnatural.

Sure, a vitamin K injection might be unnatural in the sense that our ancestors did not do it. But their babies also had higher rates of deadly bleeding, as well as the brain damage that even nonfatal bleeding can cause. Parents refusing a possibly lifesaving intervention for their newborn is likely wrapped up in growing mistrust of physicians and fear of injections. Parents who refuse the vitamin K shot are more likely to refuse routine childhood vaccinations later.

For doctors, these sorts of refusals can literally keep us up at night. I have lost track of how many times I have returned home after a day of clinic upset that I could not convince a patient to take a vaccine. Since doctors so frequently deal with poor quality data when making decisions, our rare examples of high quality data, like the safety profile and overwhelming net benefits of vaccines, matter that much more to us.

Still, I believe people who refuse vaccinations or the vitamin K injection for their baby are also making what they think is a logical decision. Let's use the vitamin K injection as an example. A mother obviously wants to protect her newborn, and may rationally feel skeptical about letting some stranger inject it with a substance she does not fully understand, for a rare complication she has never heard of before. A generation ago, that mother would have no choice except to talk to her doctor about her fears. But now, information is a quick search away online, which can easily result in her finding websites filled with low quality information or outright misinformation. The problem is, misinformation is very good at being convincing, especially when it confirms initial misgivings.

To put myself in the position of a curious mother, I tried searching "vitamin K injection at birth side effects" online. In just the first page of results, I encountered two medical sites with seemingly conflicting answers. One explains that vitamin K can theoretically lead to "severe (sometimes fatal) allergic reactions when given by injection." The other states that "there are no side effects." As a doctor, I can appreciate that these two sites are stating two different but very true things. The vitamin K injection has an extraordinarily safe side effect profile across decades of use, hence the website stating there are no side effects. If babies were regularly having allergic reactions to vitamin K, doctors would of course not be using it to prevent bleeding. But doctors and medical researchers also need to think about the risks of any intervention, so the other site claiming that there is a theoretical chance of an allergic reaction is not necessarily wrong.

Of course, a hesitant mother might find these differing takes frightening, and then find solace in the anti-vitamin K, anti-vaccination site that also comes up on the very first page of results. This site will tell her half-truths, like the vitamin K in the injection being different from vitamin K in food. It then adds that a large dose of 'synthetic' vitamin K has been linked to cancer. As a more natural alternative, it suggests eating leafy vegetables high in vitamin K in the weeks before delivery, and then breastfeeding after delivery to ensure the baby will have enough vitamins to prevent bleeding.

One thing I think doctors fail to understand about patients who act against medical advice is that, in their minds, they are acting rationally. The antiscience site did not tell the mother that her doctor was wrong, and that vitamin K was unnecessary. Instead, it told her that the medical way to treat low vitamin K had concerning side effects, and that the needed vitamin K could also be delivered in a more natural way. After reading this information, why wouldn't a skeptical mother refuse a vitamin K shot for her newborn?

A little more searching would start to poke holes in the concerns brought up by the antiscience site. The vitamin K formulation in the injection is synthetically made, but it has the same chemical structure and formula as the vitamin K you can find in spinach and other leafy vegetables. Decades ago, there were some concerns about the possibility of an association between the injection and an increased risk for cancer, but further detailed study has shown no link. And while mom can try to eat more vitamin K during pregnancy, there is, unfortunately, poor transfer of vitamin K through the placenta, meaning this strategy is ineffective. Similarly, babies obtain little vitamin K through breastfeeding.

The problem arises when the mother's doctor tries to convince her that the vitamin K injection is a good idea by calling it safe and effective, and explaining how all the newborns they have given it to have not had any issues. The doctor thinks they are addressing her concern about side effects, but by researching the issue online, the mother has already made up her mind. Moreover, the website taught her that she can avoid the issue the doctor is addressing just by eating foods rich in vitamin K before delivery. The information is wrong, but it sounds just sensible enough to give her a reason for refusal.

Doctors and patients also tend to fight over dietary supplements. Patients have easy access to websites telling them that everything from fish oil and garlic to gingko and ginseng are either age-old cures for common ailments or powerful compounds that can help them live longer.

This internet information is not necessarily wrong. Lots

of commonly taken supplements do have medical effects. There is some evidence that fish oil supplementation can improve triglyceride levels and reduce the risk of heart attacks. Plenty of doctors recommend fish oil supplements for this reason. But leading trials disagree, and the exact link between fish oil supplements and cardiovascular health is still hotly debated. Garlic lowers blood sugar levels, and gingko may help prevent memory decline in patients with Alzheimer disease. But again, evidence is mixed, trials disagree on the exact effects, and the proper dose to use, if any, is unclear. New medications have to go through extensive testing to determine safety, efficacy, dosing, and interactions with other drugs. Supplements do not have these regulations.

Let's look into one supplement, resveratrol, in a little more depth. Resveratrol is a natural compound found in grape skins as well as seeds. Proponents argue it can stop both the development and progression of cancer, in addition to having anti-inflammatory and cardioprotective effects. Multiple studies show that rodents taking resveratrol are less likely to develop cancer, seemingly proving the claims. Small human trials have also been performed, including one trial that concluded resveratrol supplementation improved cognitive performance. No wonder that resveratrol's potential benefits were the focus of a 60 Minutes special, with a leading resveratrol researcher explaining that viewers should expect the Food and Drug Administration (FDA) to approve a resveratrol-based pill within 5 years.

The problem? That 60 Minutes special aired in 2009. At the time of this writing, resveratrol is still only available in supplement form, not as a drug approved by the FDA. Opposing studies have questioned how or even if resveratrol works in humans. There is still no approved or generally recommended dose, and trials have experimented with doses ranging from just five milligrams a day up to 5,000 milligrams a day. Because resveratrol has not gone through the large, well-designed human trials required for new medications to be approved by the FDA, we lack concrete data on resveratrol's possible benefits.

I did not choose resveratrol to discuss in depth just to criticize the data behind it. On the contrary, I sincerely hope that resveratrol and compounds like it undergo further testing and are shown to be both safe and efficacious in humans. But unfortunately, a smattering of trials in mice, plus small human trials, are simply not enough data to recommend that everyone start taking a supplement. For resveratrol, and many other supplements like it, initial excitement has not been followed up by enough data. I would love to be able to give my patients a pill that delivers all the health benefits ascribed to resveratrol. But before recommending such a pill, I have to know that it actually works.

So, should you be taking vitamins and supplements? While doctors recommend vitamins in specific groups like expectant mothers and individuals who have had certain types of weight-loss surgery, there is no national recommendation for vitamin supplementation. Some studies have shown small beneficial effects of a daily multivitamin, but not every study agrees. That being said, there is no shortage of people rushing out to buy everything from a simple daily multivitamin to exotic, unproven supplements. My take is that some doctors are a bit overly dismissive, treating everything as snake oil until proven otherwise. St. John's Wort, for example, is treated as a supplement in the United States. But in Germany it is a licensed medication shown to have similar effectiveness against depression as the medications more frequently used in the U.S.

Still, at the same time, I am extremely skeptical of sources pushing overhyped, poorly tested supplements on patients. In general, I think we should put the pill bottle down, and maybe pick up a fruit or vegetable instead.

CHAPTER 7: MEDICAL EVIDENCE

WHY GOOD DATA IS SO HARD TO COME BY

By now, I sincerely hope you have learned a few things from reading this book. But I also acknowledge that one of the takeaways may be a little disheartening, that straightforward answers in medicine are far from common. Sure, doctors can confidently tell you that eating well and being active are healthy choices, but plenty of people without a medical degree know that too. I have yet to have a patient ask me "Hey doc, do you think a daily walk is healthier than eating chips on the sofa?" People already know the basics of healthy decisions without talking to a doctor. But once the questions get a little harder, like "how can I sleep better?" or "should I take a multivitamin?", the answers become increasingly more complex. There is plenty of conflicting evidence out there, often of varying levels of quality, that doctors have to wade through in order to give recommendations. Sure, guidelines can help give easy answers, but they also simplify a more complicated pool of evidence underneath.

Let's say a patient asks "Should I take a vitamin D supplement?" What is the right answer for me to give? Some doctors would look at the evidence and conclude that a large segment of the population is vitamin D deficient. And since vitamin D deficiency is associated with a lot of symptoms and diseases, it probably would not hurt to recommend a supplement. Other doctors might disagree, noting that, in the general population, vitamin D supplements have been found to have little to no benefit across many studies. And since there is both a cost and theoretical risks associated with taking any supplement, they should recommend against it. Still other doctors might leave the decision up to the patient. Are any of these doctors wrong? All of them are thinking through the available evidence, and all have their patient's best interests in mind.

This example also assumes that every doctor is completely up to date with the latest literature on vitamin D. But when doctors deal with hundreds of different clinical questions every day, it is impossible to be an expert on everything. Some doctors may simply defer to the guidelines if they feel they are not an expert on any particular topic. And regardless of the doctor's level of expertise, a true explanation of the evidence would include words like 'may,' 'suggest,' and 'likely.' Patients understandably want a simple answer, and doctors hate having to use these weasel words. And yet, very few things in medicine have crystal clear evidence behind them, and almost any intervention has some level of side effects. Even guidelines tend to rate the quality of the evidence behind the guideline, admitting that recommendations are not perfect.

As annoying as all of these complexities are, understanding them is crucial to making informed decisions, both for doctors and for patients. After all, when we fail to question the quality of evidence behind certain claims, we can end up giving or receiving unsound medical advice. There are a lot of ways certain drugs, interventions, and supplements can sound attractive based on limited evidence, even if they are ultimately useless, or even harmful.

To demonstrate the need for robust evidence, let me introduce you to a revolutionary new dietary supplement I have formulated to help with weight loss. This dietary supplement is not real, in fact it is nothing more than a simple cube of sugar. But without high-quality evidence, even a sugar pill can seem like a miracle drug.

First, because my sugar pill is a supplement, I can pretty much put it on the shelf right away. While the FDA heavily regulates new drugs coming on the market, the FDA does not approve supplements based on safety and effectiveness. In fact, the FDA must show that an already-marketed supplement is unsafe before it can be removed from the shelves. This is one of the reasons why doctors are heavily skeptical of many supplements. But for our purposes, it means that I can market my product with claims like "low-calorie" and "tastes great" without regulatory interference. After all, I am not lying. One small sugar pill really is low-calorie. If this sounds ridiculous, realize that Tic Tac® mints, which are largely flavored sugar, are able to advertise on their nutrition label that the mints have zero grams of sugar. How is this allowed? Well, since the mints are so small and the serving size is just one, the sugar content rounds down to zero, even if the mint is not sugar-free. The FDA allows this, although they did write a strongly worded letter asking companies to stop abusing sugar-free claims.

After my sugar pill supplement has been successfully marketed, and people start to buy it, let's assume that I want to run a study seeing if it has been effective. To complete this study, I randomly call up 500 people who bought the supplement, asking them to compare how hungry they felt before and after taking the supplement. When I tally up the results, I find that, on average, people felt significantly less hungry after taking the supplement. Thrilled, I then decide to add a claim on my supplement's packaging stating that it is "associated with decreased hunger in a recent study."

Wait a second, you should be screaming. That study could have simply been measuring a placebo effect. Plus, just because people felt less hungry right after taking the supplement does not mean that they will go on to lose weight. Those objections are completely valid, but real life doctors have fallen prey to similar mistakes in judgment. Vertebroplasty, a procedure used to treat back pain due to degeneration of the spine from aging or osteoporosis, was commonly performed for years. Data showed that patients felt better after the surgery than they did before, just like the people taking my mock supplement felt decreased hunger. But again, there was no placebo control. When scientists studied the procedure against a 'sham' surgery where a surgeon pretended to do the procedure but omitted key steps, there was no difference between the sham procedure and the real thing. Studies on just how effective vertebroplasty is have continued, and some people still argue it has its uses. Still, if you thought me giving people useless sugar pills looked bad, imagine giving people a useless surgery.

You might also question my study for automatically linking decreased hunger with weight loss. In real life, scientists call this a surrogate outcome. A great example is blood pressure.

Doctors do not treat high blood pressure just to make the numbers lower, but instead because high blood pressure can lead to an increased risk of dying from heart attacks and strokes. Since these events are relatively rare, it is a lot easier to test a new blood pressure medication by simply seeing if it lowers blood pressure rather than waiting to see if it lowers the risk of heart attacks and strokes. Relying largely on the surrogate outcome of blood pressure reduction, doctors prescribed a blood pressure medication called atenolol for decades. Eventually, however, it was shown that while atenolol was great at lowering blood pressure, it did not help patients avoid heart attacks or live longer lives.

After listening to critiques of my first sugar pill study, I decide to perform a second study, including both a control group and avoiding any surrogate outcomes. I randomly select 500 people who buy the supplement and measure their weight. I then measure their weight again after one month of taking the supplement. As a control, I randomly select 500 people who are not taking the supplement, and measure their weight. I measure their weight again after one month just like I did for the group taking the supplement. I crunch the numbers, finding that the control group averaged no weight change over the course of the experiment. The group taking the supplement, however, lost five pounds on average. Thrilled, I add "people taking this supplement lose five pounds in their first month" to my marketing. Again, I am not lying, and the FDA does not have to check this claim before I make it.

What happened? If I showed this experimental set up and results to a large enough group of people, I am sure I could convince some of them to buy my supplement. They would even have a relatively convincing study to demonstrate to their friends that they are following good research. But since we know this is only a sugar pill, let me offer an alternative explanation. If people in my control group were simply random people I found on the street, they probably were not trying to lose any weight. As such, their weight did not change when it was measured again a month later. But the group interested in the supplement was interested because they were trying to lose weight. Completely independent of the supplement, they made changes to lose weight, and on average lost five pounds. My sugar pill was associated with weight loss, but most certainly did not cause it.

In this example, it is pretty easy to assume that a block of sugar would not cause people to lose five pounds, but in real life, differentiating cause from effect can be extraordinarily difficult. Scientists and doctors are taught that the best way to prove causation is through a blinded, randomized-controlled trial. This means that the test group and the control group are randomly selected, but participants do not know which group they are in. The control group receives a placebo, both to keep them in the dark about being in the control group and to eliminate any possible placebo effect.

Since the placebo in the trial for my sugar pill supplement would likely be another sugar pill, this high-quality trial design would most likely conclude what we knew to be the case all along: that the sugar pill is ineffective as a weight loss supplement. But even randomized-controlled trials can still have false positive and false negative results. If twenty different research groups all around the world did high-quality studies on my supplement, it is entirely possible that one of them would report positive findings. And just as importantly, running these sorts of trials takes time. A new lifesaving treatment can spend years in trials, even as people who could benefit from it die waiting for study results.

Clearly, it is extraordinarily difficult to produce high-quality evidence proving that a new treatment actually helps patients. Conversely, my hypothetical sugar pill supplement highlights how shaky evidence can be used to make misleading claims sound convincing. Laissez-faire regulations allow many products to be advertised and sold with dubious health claims. Once people actually buy a product, the placebo effect can convince them that it is working, even if it is as useless as a sugar pill or sham surgery. Low-quality or cherry-picked studies can give a false impression that the product works much better than it actually does.

This barrage of low quality information makes it possible for marketers to sell useless placebos, bad actors to make false claims about proven vaccines, and even for the medical community to recommend useless treatments for years. What can be done to solve these problems? Personally, I believe that the issue needs to be targeted on three levels: the government, the medical and scientific fields, and finally individuals themselves. After all, we all have a role to play in ensuring that well-researched advice gets shared, and misinformation is stopped.

Let's start with what the government can do. Here, the resolution lies largely with better targeted regulations. Not only do loose regulations around the marketing of supplements allow supplement makers to get away with questionable claims, but they also mean that the product itself might not be what customers think they are getting. Independent tests have shown that many fish oil supplements on the shelves are actually rancid, with flavoring added to mask the rancid taste. Other supplements, upon independent testing, have been found to contain chemicals not on the label, including banned and potentially dangerous compounds. The lack of quality and consistency, tacitly tolerated through loose regulations, puts the health of millions of people who take supplements at risk.

Similarly, I believe direct-to-consumer advertising of medications and supplements should be more heavily regulated. Only the United States and New Zealand allow for this form of advertising, which allows pharmaceutical companies to make product claims about prescription medications to patients. Is a city billboard or thirty second TV advertisement really the best place to make claims about the evidence base behind a certain medication?

At least drug companies are marketing evidence-backed claims. The internet is awash with misinformation, and as we learned in the last chapter, it is not hard to find. As part of a broader push to counter antiscience, I would recommend that government organizations partner with technology and social media companies to keep misinformation off our feeds and search results.

While healthcare reform policies remain incredibly controversial, more needs to be done to increase Americans' access to healthcare. 25% of American adults report not having access to primary care, and the fraction of Americans without a primary care provider has been increasing in recent years. When people lack easy access to primary care, they lose access to regular checkups and preventive health screenings. But arguably just as important, they lose access to the high-quality medical information and advice that a primary care provider offers. Left with the lower-quality information and outright misinformation they might find online, these individuals are at risk of making dangerous decisions based on bad data.

Finally, the government should invest more in clinical trials. Large, randomized-controlled trials are expensive to run, which serves as a major impediment to these high-quality study designs. But because of the cost, many potentially illuminating trials are delayed for years or never run at all. As a result, doctors and scientists often face lingering controversies about best practices, and new drugs and treatments can languish for decades before approval. Public-private partnerships, as well as financial assistance, helped vaccines against COVID-19 be developed, tested, and approved all in less than a year. Similar partnerships helped battle AIDS, speeding the delivery of lifesaving treatments. But it should not take a crisis to spur these rapid advancements. If there are important questions about the efficacy of everything from flossing to resveratrol, why are we not running more clinical trials to find the answers?

The medical and scientific fields like to hold themselves up as infallible defenders of the scientific method. However, changing recommendations on everything from who should take aspirin to how frequently women should have mammograms demonstrate that medical evidence is hardly concrete. In 2013, researchers examined just one scientific journal to count the number of published studies over a period of ten years that overturned established medical practice. These changes in guidance, like vertebroplasty being found to be no better than a placebo, are known as medical reversals. How many examples could they find in just one medical journal? The answer: 146.

Conducting more high-quality trials before widespread implementation of any new medical practice can help prevent medical reversals, increasing the quality of evidence available as well as the public's trust in the scientific community. When reversals happen, scientists and doctors need to do a better job of communicating both the reasons behind the reversal, as well as what the new guidance is. Scientists and doctors also need to be more careful of discussing preliminary studies done only in cells and mouse models. A drug may seem like a miracle cure in mice, only to fail in human trials. But when scientists become overly excited about these early-stage trials, only to be met with later-stage failures, it sets the stage for increased distrust of the scientific and medical communities.

Just like any field, science and medicine are filled with people who occasionally disagree. As a result, different experts often have different opinions, even when looking at the same evidence. However, the public can easily become confused, and even distrustful, when opposing opinions are shared as absolute facts. To mitigate ill-effects of conflicting opinions, scientists and doctors must work hard to acknowledge legitimate controversies and present opinions as nothing more than personal takes. In practice, this looks like including a discussion of studies that disagree with experimental findings or personal beliefs, both in scientific publications and when talking to the lay media.

The fields of science and medicine attract a fair share of individuals with large egos, so how can we better separate opinion from fact? Thankfully, the scientific literature abounds with meta-analyses (studies combining the results of multiple smaller studies that may have come to differing conclusions) and expert reviews that consider differing viewpoints of the available evidence. By citing a consensus opinion from these analyses and reviews before offering one's personal take, scientists and doctors can give their fields greater credibility. This book, for example, relies heavily on meta-analyses and expert reviews in my attempt to avoid cherry picking data. Poor, one-sided interpretations of otherwise good science can be just as damaging as outright misinformation.

Of course, we all ultimately carry personal responsibility for not falling prey to bad information. One way we can do so is by reacting to scientific and medical news with skepticism.

Companies have a vested interest in selling us medications and supplements regardless of whether or not they will actually improve our health. Online sources can be written by anyone and filled with misinformation, even if there are links to real scientific studies. And just because something makes mice live longer does not mean it will automatically extend the lifespan of humans. I could conduct a nice, high-quality study proving that mice live longer in cat free environments. But you would laugh at me if I then suggested to outlaw pet cats for human health.

The 'ask your doctor' part of every drug commercial sounds blindingly obvious, but you might be surprised at how many patients make medical decisions without consulting their doctor. Still, in addition to just speaking with a doctor, I encourage patients to ask about the evidence and guidelines behind their doctor's recommendations. Patients should know if their physician's advice is just an opinion, and should understand if there are other options a different doctor might recommend. The best doctors are able to provide all of this information, putting ego aside to instead focus on evidence.

Finally, patients should enroll in clinical trials that they are eligible for. All those trials I would like the government to incentivize cannot actually happen if people are unwilling to participate in them. Many people are skeptical to participate in trials, and there are good historical reasons for this skepticism. Most famously, in the Tuskegee Syphilis Study, rural African American men with longstanding syphilis were not treated with antibiotics that could have cured their disease, despite antibiotics being readily available for the treatment of syphilis by the study's end. Even today, many people cite the Tuskegee study as reason to avoid enrolling in studies, expressing fears that they will be experimented on.

But today, patients participating in clinical trials are

both better informed and better protected than they were decades ago. Trials must be rigorously reviewed for safety and equity concerns before being approved, and potential subjects are fully aware of the risks and benefits of participating. While we cannot erase the stain of misguided experimentation from decades ago, we can promise patients that clinical trials today are safe, heavily-regulated ways to advance science and medicine for everyone. Instead of impassive doctors treating humans like lab rats, clinical trials run a little bit like jury duty: somewhat inconvenient and filled with paperwork, but an important part of a modern society.

Whether it is cherry-picked claims, misrepresented studies, or simply straight up misinformation, there is a lot of bad evidence out there. The Internet makes it seem like just linking to a scientific study is all that it takes to establish scientific credibility, facilitating the spread of questionable evidence. At the same time, generating high-quality evidence is extremely time-consuming and costly, meaning that dubious sources are often the easiest to find. For scientists and doctors, this leads to medical questions and controversies in the face of conflicting data. For individuals, it means wading through a steady stream of exaggerations and pseudoscience. There are ways to increase the quantity and spread of high-quality evidence, but doing so will require effort and cooperation from the government, the medical and scientific communities, and individuals. I hope we are up to the challenge.

CHAPTER 8: MEDICAL MYTHS AND CONTROVERSIES

WHY EVERYONE HAS A COMMON COLD CURE

The common cold may be common, but it also can be quite miserable. Some people are able to push through mild symptoms, but others find themselves in bed for days. And even though there are products marketed to relieve cold symptoms, anyone who has suffered through a bad cold knows a couple over-the-counter pills will not magically bring you back to normal. Not surprisingly, a lot of commonly used medications for the cold have limited benefits. Nasal decongestants like pseudoephedrine, which are extraordinarily popular as common cold treatments, were only found to reduce symptoms by 4% over the course of a typical cold. No one goes to the doctor looking for a pill that will make them feel 4% better. Similarly, evidence for common anti-cough treatments is mixed, and honey might just be as useful at stopping an annoying cough as over-the-counter medications.

These over-the-counter cold pills are in pretty much every pharmacy in the world, making it disturbing that we do not have better data on their effectiveness. At the same time, it seems like many of the people I talk to swear by their home 'cures' for the common cold. One woman proudly explained to me that she would drink a cup of tea with added ginger every day she had cold symptoms, and her concoction could magically clear up a cold in three days. I did not have the heart to tell her that, even without the tea, many cold symptoms start to disappear after three days anyway.

Regardless of the actual effectiveness of individual cold remedies, the mental connections between what we do to treat a cold and our symptoms improving are strong. In the chapter on vitamins and supplements, we discussed that while many people believe that vitamin C is a powerful anti-cold treatment, most of the evidence shows that vitamin C is hardly a miracle cure. At the same time, people who argue that vitamin C has been proven to be useless are ignoring some studies where it has slightly improved symptoms.

The other common cold treatment that stirs up nearly as much controversy as vitamin C is zinc. Zinc preparations have been shown to reduce the duration of the common cold, but only with a high enough dose of zinc. However, side effects such as taste changes and nausea are associated with zinc supplementation, making researchers question if the side effects are worse than a few extra hours of cold symptoms. A possible link between intranasal zinc sprays and permanent loss of smell spurred the FDA to specifically warn consumers against trying these products. Contrary to popular belief, supplements can have pernicious side effects.

Cautious supplementation with vitamin C and oral zinc lozenges is not pseudoscience, even though many doctors are rightfully skeptical of these treatments due to their limited benefits and notable side effects. That being said, skeptical physicians might want to turn some of their distrust toward their own profession. Many doctors incorrectly prescribe antibiotics, which only treat bacterial infections and not the viruses that cause the common cold, to patients with common cold symptoms. One study found that a shocking 46% of patients with a viral infection were still given antibiotics. Older and busier doctors, on average, were more likely to hand out these incorrect prescriptions. Beyond potentially leading to antibiotic resistance and side effects, these prescriptions offer no clinical benefit to the patient.

Inappropriate antibiotic prescriptions from doctors aside, I tend to give people lots of leeway for their at-home common cold cures, regardless of their proven efficacy. Chicken noodle soup may not be proven to shorten cold symptoms, but if it feels good on a sore throat, then why not have some? When I have a cold, my personal solution to minimize symptoms is taking frequent, hot showers. I find this provides me some temporary relief. However, evidence from a randomized-controlled trial argues that steam inhalation, the main point behind me taking these hot showers, may not improve cold symptoms. Still, just like many of my patients, I have decided to stick with my personal common cold 'cure,' regardless of the weak evidence behind it in the scientific literature.

When diagnosing patients with the common cold, doctors are stuck with few options for effective treatment. Luckily, patients with influenza can be prescribed oseltamivir, an antiviral medication that is effective against the flu. But oseltamivir (more commonly known by the brand name Tamiflu) is itself controversial. A large review of oseltamivir studies found that, on average, oseltamivir shortens flu symptoms in adults by 17 hours. On one hand, shortening symptoms by less than a day is not a huge benefit. But on the other hand, having the flu is a miserable experience, and moving the symptoms along, even if just by a few hours, can mean a big deal for patients. Of course, oseltamivir is not without its possible side effects, including headache, nausea, damage to kidneys, and an increased risk of psychiatric events. Doctors have to compare these risks against the possible benefits before recommending the treatment to patients. Since the benefits of oseltamivir seem to decrease the longer symptoms persist before treatment, prescribing oseltamivir to patients who have been symptomatic for two or more days may expose them to the risk of side effects without any benefit in shortening symptoms.

Myths and controversies about these common illnesses abound, but the cold and flu viruses are not the only topic of debate. Ever been told that you need to drink eight glasses of water every day? One researcher tried to determine where the rule came from, only to find no clear origin and no evidence to back it up. Below, I outline other controversial health topics frequently brought up by my patients in clinic as well as by family and friends.

The 10,000 Step Rule

A generation ago, asking a friend "how many steps did you walk yesterday?" would be more likely to merit a confused look than an actual answer. Who would care about, or be able to count up, their exact number of steps? But after a pedometer craze in the early 2000s, knowing how many steps you had walked by the end of the day became common. Now, with smartphones in our pockets at all hours, not to mention many people with additional wearable fitness trackers, we are more in tune of our step count than ever before.

It has become a tenet of step counting that averaging 10,000 steps a day is a healthy goal. Many wearable fitness trackers have pushed users to hit a daily 10,000 step target. The American Heart Association suggests walkers work their way up to 10,000 steps, and the same step goal has also been used to increase physical activity in clinical trials. But is there something special about the number 10,000 specifically?

Interestingly, there is something special about the number 10,000, but not in the way you may think. Far from being a tenet of physical fitness, the original inspiration for the 10,000 step goal is really just a Japanese pun, as the Japanese character for 10,000 looks a bit like a walking figure. When pedometers become popular in 1960s Japan, marketers took advantage of this clever pun. These "10,000 steps meters," literally translating the Japanese title into English, became popular in other countries, spreading the concept of taking 10,000 steps per day around the world.

Just because 10,000 steps is a relatively arbitrary goal does not mean that we should ignore it. After all, Americans are notoriously sedentary, with one survey finding that people barely averaged 5,000 steps a day. There is good evidence suggesting people who take more steps are healthier. A separate study found that the more steps someone walked on average, the less likely they were to die over the study's follow-up period. And even just having a target number of steps to hit seems like it can motivate physical activity, as numerous studies have shown that tracking one's daily steps leads to an increase in steps taken. Ultimately, merely having a goal might be more important than hitting any arbitrary number. A study looking at older women found a significantly decreased risk of mortality for women averaging just 4,400 steps a day compared to their less active counterparts, who averaged 2,700 steps a day. Mortality rates decreased as the daily step count increased, but the benefits seemed to level off around 7,500 steps per day, much lower than the 10,000 step recommendation. Of course, these findings should not encourage younger adults, who should be more mobile than their older neighbors, to simply stop their daily activity at 4,400 or even 7,500 steps.

Stretching

Flexibility training was notably absent from our discussion of physical activity in the chapter on exercise. Unlike aerobic training and strength training, the Physical Activity Guidelines for Americans do not include any recommendations for stretching or other flexibility exercises. Yet, many people still swear by stretching before and after their workouts. Does stretching work? The answer is surprisingly complex. As you might expect, stretching has been shown to increase range of motion, meaning that it can help make you more flexible. If your only goal is to be able to touch your toes, then developing a stretching regimen to reach that goal makes perfect sense. That being said, flexibility is not the only claimed benefit of stretching. Advocates also claim that it can improve performance, reduce the risk of injury, and decrease pain after a workout.

Let's tackle performance first. One review paper, summarizing multiple studies, found that stretching before an activity slightly decreased athletic performance on average, with bigger impacts on performance the longer the stretch was held. Different experts, writing a review paper of their own, also acknowledged that some studies showed negative results on athletic performance from static stretching. However, they also called attention to studies finding no performance changes after stretching as well as studies, especially after dynamic stretching, that showed improved performance.

What is the source of the controversy? Well, one issue is that there are lots of different kinds of stretches. Beyond dividing stretching into static versus dynamic stretches, researchers also have to consider how intense the stretch is as well as how long the stretch is held for. The definition of performance is also vague. Increased performance can mean running a faster mile, jumping higher, or lifting more weight, depending on the study. But these different activities require very different kinds of efforts from our muscles, complicating matters further. It is very possible that some stretching might help a runner's performance while being a net negative for a weightlifter, for instance.

Adding to the controversy, an analysis of over 5,000 individuals found no significant decrease in running injuries in runners who completed stretches as a part of their workout. Admittedly, one negative study does not mean that stretching is completely useless, as different stretching regimens and different definitions of what counts as a running injury could have affected these findings. But stretching enthusiasts looking for strong data to support the common assertion that stretching can prevent injuries will be disappointed. On the contrary, studies have shown that stretching before, after, or both before and after a workout will not reduce the risk of developing delayed onset muscle soreness.

All this data, in my opinion, does not mean that stretching is a hoax. Sports coaches who advocate mandatory stretching to prevent injury are doing so without clear evidence, but it is not a secret that a lot of athletes simply prefer to stretch before a workout or competition. If the process of stretching makes them feel more limber and mentally prepared, then it might be worth the time spent.

Superfoods

I cannot specifically recall ever hearing a doctor use the term 'superfood.' And yet, articles about superfoods with miraculous health benefits are all over the internet, and the word has snuck into the popular lexicon. My mother, whose lunch is commonly a medley of grapes, strawberries, and blueberries eaten with yogurt, will proudly tell you that her blueberries are a superfood. Admittedly, she is not wrong. Berries have been shown to have powerful effects like improving insulin sensitivity and decreasing cholesterol levels. But just because blueberries are commonly listed as a superfood and grapes, for example, are not always included, does not magically make blueberries a much healthier choice.

In general, I admire the concept of trying to entice people to pick out healthy foods. But I have two issues with the concept of singling out specific superfoods. First, as I have already made clear, superfoods appear to be somewhat arbitrarily selected. Kale, another frequent entrant on superfood lists, is undoubtedly a healthy choice. But experts in nutrition, writing a review of kale's benefits, still made sure to note it is "unclear why kale is declared superior" to similar leafy greens. When I discuss healthy eating choices with patients, I am not too concerned about whether they choose to eat kale or spinach. I just want them to be eating something green. There are plenty of healthy options out there that are not necessarily listed as 'super.'

The other issue I have with superfoods is that they can seem inaccessible to the average person. One barrier to superfoods is their cost. Fruit does not have to be expensive, but a serving of blueberries is generally much more expensive than an apple or a banana. Wealthier individuals are much more likely to eat some of the more exotic superfoods like quinoa, goji berries, and wheatgrass. After all, these foods can be quite expensive. As such, superfoods can make healthy eating seem to be synonymous with expensive eating, which does not necessarily need to be the case. If someone only has $1 to spend on a snack, a $4 serving of goji berries does not do them any good. But choosing the $1 apple over the $1 bag of chips is a much healthier option. Healthy food does not need to be super; it just needs to be accessible.

Organics and GMOs

Most people have a general idea that organic food is healthier than non-organic food, but may not be able to come up with a specific definition of what organic actually means. Thankfully, the U.S. Department of Agriculture (USDA) uses a strict set of rules to certify foods as being organic. Under the USDA's definition, produce is organic if it is grown on soil free from prohibited substances, notably synthetic pesticides and fertilizers. Meat can be organic if the animals are given adequate room to graze, eat organic feed, and are allowed to grow without hormones or antibiotics. These definitions matter when buying individual ingredients like chicken or an eggplant. But organic labels pop up on more processed, multi-ingredient foods as well. Here, the labelling gets tricky. If 95% or more of the food comes from organic materials, the food can be labelled as organic, with a USDA organic seal. If between 70 and 95% of the food is organic, the food can only be labelled as being made with organic ingredients. Long story short: organic has a definition, but context clearly matters.

Are organic foods actually healthier? Well, it depends what you mean when you say healthier. Organic foods do not appear to be more nutritious than non-organic foods. This means that if you are looking for more vitamins or minerals through buying organic, you are not getting any benefits for your money. However, organic foods do contain less pesticide residues than non-organic alternatives. If you are concerned about these products in your food, then organic options make a lot of sense. Of course, the actual health consequences of trace amounts of pesticides are still hotly debated. People who eat organic foods regularly are, for example, less likely to be obese. That being said, it also makes sense that healthier people are the ones most likely to seek out and buy organic foods, and there are no clear causal links between an organic diet and improved clinical outcomes.

GMOs, short for genetically modified organisms, are sometimes viewed as the unhealthy opposite of organics. However, the truth is a bit more nuanced. Although modern science has accelerated the process, humans have genetically modified our food for thousands of years. Ancient farming communities would breed plants to encourage bigger yields, purposely selecting for certain traits. In a similar way, humans have genetically modified dogs, not just to make them friendlier than ancient wolves, but to select for the different features that differentiate a chihuahua from a Doberman. Unlike organics, which are not associated with higher vitamin contents, genetically modified food can actually provide extra vitamins and nutrients. For example, a strain of rice has been modified to increase its vitamin A content, potentially helping fight vitamin A deficiency in poorer nations.

There are legitimate concerns about GMOs, including the possibility for unexpected allergic reactions. There have been theoretical links between certain GMO products and unwanted side effects, like mice with disordered cell division after eating GMO potatoes. That being said, products meant for human consumption are tested for safety before entering the market, and there is no evidence that approved GMOs are causing direct harms.

My take? If you are willing to pay a little more money in exchange for less pesticide exposure, then shell out for organic. But be aware that there is no clear evidence saying that organic foods will make you healthier in the long term, and you are essentially paying for extra peace of mind. GMOs are often unfairly maligned and quite safe in practice, but their theoretical risks mean that the industry should continue to be regulated.

Keto and paleo diets

The keto diet, in which the dieter heavily restricts carbohydrate intake but is allowed relatively unrestricted access to proteins and fats, is a popular recent fad diet. As discussed in the chapter on nutrition, pretty much any diet can help you lose weight if it leads to a decrease in total calories consumed. But while the keto diet can work to help weight loss, doctors know it best as a method to decrease the risk of recurrent seizures in people with epilepsy.

Unfortunately, for those of us without epilepsy, the special benefits of the keto diet are probably limited. There is some concern that replacing carbohydrates with protein and fat could actually increase mortality in the long term. On the other hand, keto diet supporters argue that the diet could create an unfavorable environment for cancer cells. Still, these theories have not been rigorously tested, and there is no strong evidence for the long-term superiority of a keto diet.

The paleo diet, in which the dieter tries to limit foods

to those available to our hunter-gatherer ancestors, is another recent dieting fad. On the surface, the logic makes some sense. A lot of the foods we eat now, like processed sugars and salty snacks, were not available to our ancestors and lead to diseases like diabetes and hypertension. As such, adherents to the paleo diet largely limit their intake to meat, fruits, and vegetables. Grains and dairy products are frowned upon. There are some small studies showing that the paleo diet can lead to weight loss. But then again, pretty much any diet can. A review article summarizing several preliminary studies on the paleo diet says it best: the diet is currently "over-hyped and under-researched."

Marijuana

Marijuana legalization remains a controversial political topic, but there has definitely been a trend toward increasing access to both medical and recreational marijuana. I tell my patients who are curious about trying marijuana, either for a medical condition or recreationally, is that it is best to view marijuana first and foremost as a drug. Why do I say this? Because both marijuana advocates and marijuana detractors frequently use poor arguments to justify their positions. Marijuana advocates often focus on the fact that marijuana, being just a plant, is natural and therefore safe. Sure, marijuana is a plant, but so are poison ivy and hemlock. You do not see people lining up to ingest those plants just because they are natural.

Of course, marijuana detractors also overstate their case by arguing that marijuana is a dangerous, mild-altering substance, and therefore must be heavily regulated or illegal. However, the exact same arguments could be said about alcohol. The CDC estimates that alcohol is involved in almost 100,000 deaths per year, and yet drinking a beer or glass of wine does not carry the same social stigma as marijuana use.

These glaring oversimplifications ignore that, being a drug, marijuana has both intended effects and side effects, and both are important to consider before using. For recreational marijuana users, the intended effect is simply the 'high' that they are seeking. Medical marijuana users cite a variety of potential benefits. There is strong evidence that marijuana can reduce chronic pain, decrease chemotherapy-associated nausea and vomiting, and decrease muscle spasms in patients with multiple sclerosis. These are important benefits, especially considering that chronic pain affects hundreds of millions of people around the world, and is notoriously difficult to treat. Evidence for potential other benefits of marijuana is emerging, but with less clear-cut evidence. Of particular interest is the potential that marijuana can help people with mental health diagnoses like depression or PTSD, but there is only limited evidence to date on these possible benefits.

As I have made clear, every drug has its side effects, and marijuana is no exception. Some side effects are obvious, like smoking marijuana being associated with increased cough, wheezing, and shortness of breath. Slightly less obvious is the possibility of weight gain from snacking while high, as well as the possibility of increased car accidents as people under the influence of marijuana drive. Other concerning side effects include an increased risk of heart attack after smoking marijuana, as well as a connection between marijuana use and schizophrenia.

Like all drugs, I think people should look at the intended benefits, as well as the possible risks, of marijuana usage. Focusing on the medical facts and data, not the political rhetoric and controversy, is the right way to move forward. There definitely are legitimate medical applications of marijuana, and the chronic pain patients it might benefit most have long struggled with limited treatment options. Of course, like any other drug, users should be aware of its limitations and side effects.

CHAPTER 9: THE HEALTHCARE SYSTEM

WHY NINE MILES CAN CUT 30 YEARS OFF YOUR LIFE

Chicago has always been 'my city', and I chose to pursue both medical school and residency training through the University of Chicago. As any Chicagoan will proudly tell you, the most distinctive aspect of the city is its many neighborhoods. The Loop, in the center of the city, has towering office buildings and award-winning museums. Humboldt Park, on the city's northwest side, is known for its strong Puerto Rican community and signature jibarito sandwich. Hyde Park, to the south, is known for its century-old mansions and dense collection of Nobel laureates. But even with our pride for the city's many neighborhoods, Chicagoans also have to acknowledge that the neighborhood system helps underscore deep inequities within the city. It is very easy to tell a lot about a Chicagoan just from knowing where they live.

Take the neighborhood of Streeterville as an example. Just north of the Loop, Streeterville is home to the Magnificent Mile and Navy Pier. Living there, however, is quite pricey, and residents' median income is around $100,000 a year. But if you can afford it, Streeterville is the also the Chicago neighborhood with the longest life expectancy. Chicagoans in Streeterville can expect to live to 90, on average. Nine miles south of Streeterville, the neighborhood of Englewood looks very different. In stark contrast to Streeterville's towering high rises, Englewood is littered with empty lots, and many residents live below the poverty line. The median income in Englewood is $22,000. Life expectancy is just 60.

Let that sink in for a second. Residents of the two neighborhoods live in the same country, the same state, and even the same city. As such, Englewood residents theoretically have access to the same medical facilities as people in wealthier areas of the city, like Streeterville. And yet, they die 30 years earlier on average. The life expectancy gap between the two neighborhoods is the largest in the country. How did such a large gap develop?

Invoking Chicago's stereotype of gun violence to explain the life expectancy gap is an easy explanation, but it is ultimately incorrect. Yes, there are huge variations in violent crime between Chicago neighborhoods, with neighborhoods like Englewood having a homicide rate 10 times greater than some of Chicago's wealthier neighborhoods. But all in all, murder is still extremely rare, and does little to explain away a shocking 30 year gap in life expectancy. Another poor explanation for the life expectancy gap is the availability of quality healthcare. Sure, Streeterville is home to Northwestern Memorial Hospital, a highly-ranked academic hospital capable of handling the most complex patients. But the same could be said for the University of Chicago Hospital, which is just a few blocks away from Englewood.

Admittedly, the availability of healthcare does not necessarily translate to accessibility of healthcare. And this is where we start to uncover some of the bigger reasons for the life expectancy gap. While it is hard to find quality data on access to healthcare by neighborhood, it is not hard to imagine that in an impoverished area like Englewood, many residents have to decide between paying for their medicine or paying for food. Unemployed or uninsured individuals are likely to struggle to find a doctor they can afford to see, and people who are working may not have the economic flexibility to go to an appointment. Even for people who can attend their appointment and can afford their medication, limited pharmacy options in the area mean that lines to pick up a prescription can stretch out the door. Of course life expectancy is lower. Residents of Englewood face obstacles to almost every interaction with the healthcare system.

Worse, the inequities can run deeper. Beyond just their interactions with the healthcare system, Englewood residents face many other barriers to good health. Lower-quality housing is associated with increased allergy triggers in disadvantaged neighborhoods. As a result, neighborhoods like Englewood have noticeably higher rates of asthma than wealthier neighborhoods in Chicago. At the same time, Englewood residents struggle to find healthy food, both due to economic constraints and limited grocery options in the area. Limited access to healthy food fuels lifestyle diseases like diabetes and hypertension, both of which are more common in Englewood than the city as a whole. Socioeconomic disadvantages create health inequalities, then throw up barriers to healthcare access and treatment. The result: a frightening 30 year gap in life expectancy.

The Englewood example makes it seem like poverty is inextricably related to a shortened life expectancy, and that lower-income individuals face a near-impossible battle in trying to live as long as their wealthier peers. But cross-country comparisons show that this is simply not the case. The $22,000 median income in Englewood is low by American standards. But remember our fake centenarians in Vilcabama, Ecuador? They would probably love to earn that income. Per capita income in Ecuador is just $6,000. Yet, life expectancy is 77 years, closer to Streeterville than Englewood.[1] In fact, Ecuador's 77 year life expectancy is almost equal to the United States' life expectancy of 79 years, despite Ecuador being a much poorer country. This is not something magical about Ecuador. Remember, we disproved the theory that people there have some magical fountain of youth. Plenty of countries that are much poorer than the United States have life expectancies roughly equal to, or even higher than, the U.S. average.

Compared to citizens of similarly wealthy countries, Americans die younger on average, despite the American medical system spending more money trying to keep them alive. It really does not matter which wealthy country you compare the US against, the rule holds true for Switzerland, Germany, France, the United Kingdom, Canada, Australia, and New Zealand. The list could go on. The United States spends about 17 cents out of every dollar on healthcare. The average healthcare spending within the Organisation for Economic Co-operation and Development (OECD), a group of wealthy nations, is roughly half that. Meanwhile, people living in other

---

[1] Life expectancy numbers have bounced around a great deal since the start of the COVID-19 pandemic. Here, I use prepandemic data.

OECD nations live longer, healthier lives on average. And while Americans spend more and more on healthcare, we seem to be getting less and less out of our investment. U.S. life expectancy peaked in 2014. It has been trending downward ever since.

Why is there such a discrepancy between ballooning healthcare expenses and limited longevity benefits, especially when compared to other countries? The first and most obvious answer is that Americans simply pay a higher sticker price for healthcare resources. It is not a secret that American doctors tend to take home large paychecks. But the costs do not stop with us doctors. Nurses in the U.S. make more money than nurses in other wealthy nations. Insulin in the United States, literally a lifesaving medication for many, can cost ten times more in America that it does in France or the United Kingdom. This pattern repeats itself for the cost of many other drugs, leading to the U.S. spending more money per capita on pharmaceuticals than any other wealthy nation. Add in the exorbitant costs of bloodwork, X-rays, CT scans, and MRIs in the United States, and it becomes a little easier to understand how we spend trillions of dollars each year on healthcare.

That being said, high costs are not the only explanation. Americans are also less healthy on average than people in other countries. Obesity rates in the U.S. are roughly twice as high as the OECD average, and more than one in four Americans have two or more chronic diseases. These chronic diseases, like diabetes and high blood pressure, require regular medical attention to safely control. But barriers preventing Americans from accessing the healthcare system mean that these diseases are often left uncontrolled. The average American sees a doctor four times a year. The average German, in contrast, sees a doctor ten times a year. Uncontrolled disease leads to expensive complications. Metformin, a staple diabetes drug often used for people with well-controlled diabetes, is extraordinarily cheap, with a month's supply costing just a few dollars. Meanwhile, diabetic ketoacidosis, a potentially fatal complication of poorly controlled diabetes, can lead to a hospitalization costing hundreds of thousands of dollars.

Preventing someone from needing such a costly hospitalization is an obvious goal, but at least the money used to pay for that hospitalization can save a life. On the contrary, a great deal of money spent on healthcare in the U.S. seems to be completely wasted. A study published in *The Journal of the American Medical Association* tried to calculate the value of this medical waste. Their estimate: 760 billion to 935 billion dollars are wasted every year, meaning that about 25% of total U.S. healthcare spending does not help people feel better, get healthier, or live longer at all.

How can medical spending be wasted? Some causes are simple, like pharmacies charging different prices for the same medication. If someone pays $20 for a drug they could have bought for $10 across the street, that is an example of wasteful spending. But the same wasteful spending occurs on a much larger scale when insurers pay hospitals $10,000 for a procedure that could have cost only $5,000 elsewhere. Remember vertebroplasty, the surgery designed to improve back pain that ultimately turned out to be no better than a placebo in a later trial? Those surgical expenses can also be considered wasted healthcare dollars. Other inefficiencies of our healthcare system, like patients going to the emergency room for a complaint that could have been solved by their regular physician, or insurers and hospitals spending undue time and money to negotiate payments, also contribute to healthcare waste.

These problems are not necessarily unique to the American healthcare system, but together, they push our costs upward and cause us to spend significantly more than similar countries. As such, one way to better understand both the strengths and weaknesses of the American system is to educate ourselves on how other countries structure their healthcare systems. Every healthcare system is unique, but common models do stand out.

One model that the United States is often compared against is the Beveridge Model, a socialized form of healthcare best exemplified by the United Kingdom's National Health Service. Under this model, the government collects tax revenue to make healthcare a public service. Doctors, nurses, and other hospital staff are paid by the government. Similarly, healthcare clinics and hospitals are public buildings just like libraries and police stations in the United States. Canada uses a national health insurance model, where doctors and hospitals are private entities, but the government controls all insurance payouts. The Bismarck Model, invented and used in Germany, has private insurance plans as well as private doctors and hospitals, but the system is heavily regulated by the government to control prices and prevent private insurers from making large profits.

What is interesting about America is that we have failed to select one main model. For Americans with private health insurance through their employer, the American system looks a bit like Germany's, albeit with less stringent government regulations. Once people turn 65 and switch to Medicare, however, the system looks a lot like Canada's. Veterans can seek care at Veterans Affairs clinics and hospitals, which are paid for and run by the government, mirroring the UK's National Health Service. Uninsured Americans, largely excluded from any of these models, are essentially forced to pay out of pocket for healthcare.

There is an argument to be made that America's

mixture of so many different models makes the overall system less efficient. That being said, fixing the many issues with healthcare in America is not as simple as picking the single best model. Any model, if poorly implemented, can fail to provide high-quality, affordable healthcare. Policymakers can debate over which model is 'right' for America moving forward, but if recent history is any guide, a complete overhaul of the healthcare system is rather unlikely. The most recent major change, The Affordable Care Act, was a more targeted reform. Among other things, it provided insurance marketplaces and expanded Medicaid in order to give more Americans insurance.

Helping ensure that people have insurance makes a lot of sense. After all, insurance allows people to have affordable access to healthcare, which theoretically should improve overall health. But interestingly, some studies have cast doubt on this relationship. A classic experiment done by the RAND corporation in the 1970s and 1980s enrolled different families in insurance programs with different levels of coverage. The experiment found that people with less comprehensive insurance, meaning those who had to pay more out of pocket for coverage, ended up using less healthcare on average. In other words, people rationed healthcare based on the costs they would personally face. But at the end of the study, there were only minimal differences in health outcomes between people with different levels of insurance coverage. Put simply, better insurance led to more healthcare, but more healthcare did not necessarily make people healthier. A similar finding occurred when Oregon expanded Medicaid based on a lottery system, essentially creating a randomized-controlled trial for the effectiveness of Medicaid. People who now had Medicaid used more healthcare resources, but were no more likely to have lower blood pressure or better cholesterol numbers.

These two examples have been hotly debated for years by doctors, economists, and policymakers. One opinion about the results is that health insurance offers economic protection, but does not lead to improved health. Under this argument, America's recent push to expand health insurance, both through subsidized online health exchanges and Medicaid expansion, is largely a waste of money. These findings are rather shocking, especially considering that people with insurance in these studies were more likely to make doctor's appointments, more likely to go to the emergency room, and more likely to be hospitalized. This implies that all those healthcare resources, as well as the healthcare dollars used to pay for them, were essentially being wasted. Perhaps our issue with wasted spending is even more pervasive than it first seemed.

This line of thinking argues that many doctor's appointments are essentially worthless, because they fail to lead to demonstrable health benefits. But as someone who works in primary care, I have to respectfully disagree. Imagine a patient who comes in to see their doctor complaining of low back pain that started the day after they moved heavy boxes. Since acetaminophen at home did not help, they are curious if the pain will go away, and wondering if they need an X-ray or MRI. After taking a history and performing a physical exam, the doctor diagnoses them with acute muscle strain. The doctor recommends against imaging, but suggests they try over the counter ibuprofen and lidocaine patches for pain relief.

I would call this a rather typical clinic visit, but its benefits would be hard to clarify under these studies' designs. The back pain would have likely gone away on its own over several weeks, and all the doctor did was recommend medications the patient could have obtained without seeing a doctor. And yet, if the history and physical exam would have been more suggestive of a spinal fracture or nerve impingement, the doctor would have had a different treatment approach. In other words, the doctor's medical expertise was still useful, even though the patient was essentially told to let the injury heal on its own. However, a study trying to link medical care with improved outcomes could conclude that this visit did little to make the patient live a longer or healthier life.

In fact, people who received insurance under Oregon's Medicaid expansion were more likely to report that they were in good or excellent health than people who did not, even as their blood pressures and cholesterol levels remained similar. Depression rates in Medicaid enrollees were reduced 30% compared to their unenrolled counterparts. And importantly, the insurance coverage significantly reduced enrollees' risk of having to borrow money or leave bills unpaid due to medical expenses.

Another important thing to remember is that these studies measured health outcomes over years. But remember the Look AHEAD study, where individuals with diabetes received a wide variety of resources to help them lose weight? One of the lessons from that study is that lifestyle choices do matter, but it takes many years to even decades in order to observe outcomes. It is entirely possible that these studies simply did not follow people for a long enough time to see results. In Oregon, Medicaid enrollees were more likely to be both diagnosed with diabetes and receiving proper treatment than individuals who did not receive Medicaid. The mortality differences may not have been clear over the course of the study, but I know that I would much rather be treated for diabetes than not even know I had it.

America's recent major health reforms have been focused on expanding insurance coverage, and even that is controversial. What else can we be doing to improve our healthcare system? Many people have spent years advocating for large-scale changes. Looking at the current system's constellation of rising insurance premiums, millions of uninsured Americans, and families declaring bankruptcy to erase medical debt, I certainly cannot blame them. But with political gridlock complicating large scale changes, I want to focus on smaller, more immediate solutions.

First things first. If healthcare costs in America are out of control, then more should be done to rein in outrageous prices. Most newer drugs are expensive because they are still patent protected, meaning cheaper generic forms cannot legally be sold. Limiting the power of drug patents would likely lower medication costs, but it would also decrease drug companies' incentive to spend millions on the research and development process for new drugs. There is definitely a good reason to have some level of patent protection in place. Still, pharmaceutical companies, often with billions of dollars in profits and the ability to hire large teams of lawyers, are frequently able to stretch the rules of the patent protection framework. As such, there is a lot more the government could be doing to decrease drug costs, including clarifying patent protections and directly negotiating drug prices with pharmaceutical companies.

Perhaps drug prices should better reflect how much value they provide to patients. This sort of pricing is already in use within the healthcare system. In recent years, both private insurance companies and Medicare have started to tie reimbursement payments to doctors and hospitals based on the health value of the services rendered. For example, a hospital might be paid a fixed fee for a hospitalization, instead of being paid for each medication or procedure administered. These regulations incentivize hospitals and clinics to only provide care that will actually help the patient, and not just run up the bill.

Healthcare economists call this system of payment value-based care, meaning that instead of doctors receiving a flat fee for providing a particular service, they are paid based on the actual value that service provides to the patient. As a way of linking healthcare costs with patient outcomes, these value-based programs make a lot of sense. But at the same time, there are some downsides. For starters, the definition of 'value' is not always obvious. Plus, by separating specific services rendered from those services' costs, healthcare pricing may become even more convoluted. And while it makes sense to reward doctors and hospitals that are providing high value care, changing reimbursement systems will have ripple effects. Imagine a small, rural hospital that finds it can no longer stay solvent with value-based payments, even though it is the only hospital in the area. Try explaining to the surrounding communities that the reason they no longer have any local emergency room is because of new regulations.

Clearly, any changes to the healthcare system are extremely complicated. That being said, I believe a few cost-cutting measures are worth the side effects. First, I would like to see increased price transparency. Patients should not have to guess which hospital will provide a cheaper ultrasound or hip replacement. When a doctor orders bloodwork for a cost-conscious patient, they should be able to look up the expected cost before the patient leaves the clinic. Second, I would like to see stricter regulations to make insurance coverage more uniform. Under our current system, individuals switching insurances can find that their doctor is suddenly out of network, or that their prescription that used to cost $5 now costs $50 or more. Wouldn't it be nice if similar insurance plans covered the same providers, medicines, and procedures? Patients would not have to worry about surprise bills threatening their economic stability, and doctors could more confidently estimate the costs of a particular treatment. And finally, I would like to see legislation that addresses the exorbitant costs of medications. Companies should have incentives to research new drugs, but there is no reason why Americans need to pay many times more than citizens of other countries for medication. Insulin, at least, has become cheaper for many, as the Inflation Reduction Act of 2022 capped insulin costs at $35 for Medicare enrollees. While this price cap serves as a wonderful proof of concept for legislation making drugs more affordable, there are countless other needed medications that many Americans still struggle to afford.

Of course, addressing healthcare costs does not necessarily solve the issue of healthcare access. The best solution here is simple, although admittedly not immediate: we need to train more doctors. The Medicare program helps fund residency positions, allowing medical school graduates to train and specialize. But Congress has been slow to increase funding for residency positions, even as the number of medical school graduates has grown in recent years. The result is that there are medical school graduates who are unable to find residency training positions, even as the country decries a shortage of doctors.

More doctors does not necessarily mean more access to general healthcare if all of them decide to become dermatologists or spine surgeons. Primary care doctors tend to make far less money than specialists, driving medical school graduates away from primary care as a specialty. But at the same time, millions of Americans lack a primary care doctor, and even those who can afford an appointment are often disappointed with the long wait to see a physician. A solution here is to offer additional compensation to primary care doctors to incentivize more doctors to think twice about picking a niche specialty. More Federally Qualified Health Centers, which receive special funds to offer low-cost care in underserved areas, could also help increase access to primary care physicians. Sure, there are costs associated with increasing primary care compensation and subsidizing safety net clinics. However, I like to view these costs as investments. After all, primary care appointments cost the healthcare system far less than the ER visits and hospitalizations that accrue as patients cannot control their chronic medical conditions without adequate primary care.

Not every fix is easy. I would love an easy way to make the population more fit, so that we can save money on treating the many complications associated with obesity. Some localities have experimented with taxing sugary drinks, and these taxes have been successful in reducing soft drink consumption. However, proposals to tax soda generate enormous controversy, and soft drink consumption is far from the only unhealthy behavior. In other words, we could ban soda entirely, but Americans would still be just as obese if they traded sugary drinks for sugary snacks instead.

Healthcare policy proposals in general are complex, controversial, and unlikely to solve every issue our healthcare system faces. However, we cannot let these obstacles to meaningful change stop us from trying to make the healthcare system more accessible and more cost-effective. When poor Americans are dying decades earlier than their wealthy counterparts, the system is clearly broken. It is up to us to figure out how we want to fix it.

CHAPTER 10: PREVENTIVE MEDICINE

WHY A WELLNESS VISIT IS MORE COMPLICATED THAN YOU THINK

Preventive medicine makes a lot of sense. Instead of treating injuries or diseases once they happen, we can try to prevent them from happening in the first place. At the most basic level, this means eating a healthy diet, maintaining a normal weight, exercising regularly, and not smoking. This sounds like easy, sensible advice to follow. And yet, as a country, we do a terrible job of following these recommendations. Our poor diets lead to weight gain, resulting in an appalling 74% of American adults being either overweight or obese. We've already discussed that less than 25% of Americans meet the government's rather modest goal for physical activity. And despite decades of work to lower smoking rates, 14% of adult Americans still smoke. All in all, only a relatively small fraction of Americans actually follow the basic tenets for healthy living.

The irony is that even as Americans fail to eat well and exercise frequently, we do a pretty good job of lining up for screening tests like colonoscopies, pap smears, and mammograms. While screening rates could always improve, between 60% and 80% of Americans undergo these tests as recommended. Our relatively high rates are cause for celebration, as cancer screening tests are literal lifesavers. For example, having a colonoscopy reduces the risk of dying from colorectal cancer by about two thirds. Even with screening tests being commonplace, roughly 50,000 Americans die from colorectal cancer yearly, implying that colonoscopies save tens of thousands of American lives every year.

Clearly, colon cancer screening is a good idea. It earns an "A" rating from the United States Preventive Services Task Force. The U.S. Preventive Services Task Force is perhaps the most famous creator of guidelines for preventive health, and their "A" rating indicates there is strong evidence for substantial benefit to patients. But even though colonoscopies save tens of thousands of lives yearly, those lives pale in comparison to the amount of lives lost each year from heart disease (697,000), strokes (160,000), and diabetes (102,000). All of these causes of death are linked quite closely to our lifestyle choices. The point here: get your colonoscopy, but realize that a healthy lifestyle is even more important. I cannot emphasize this enough. If we could spend all the money used to provide colonoscopies, pap smears, and mammograms, and instead direct it to eliminate obesity, we would save hundreds of thousands more lives each year.

So, why don't we? Unfortunately, lifestyle changes are hard to implement, and having a conversation with someone about healthy eating will not necessarily lead to weight loss.

When a doctor preforms a colonoscopy, they can be pretty sure their patient does not have colon cancer. But when a doctor counsels a patient on weight loss, that patient can very easily come back to their next appointment having not lost a pound. Counseling patients on weight loss and lifestyle changes can still improve outcomes, but if all it took to cure obesity was a simple doctor's visit, America would not be suffering an obesity crisis. Instead, doctors focus so much on cancer screening tools because they are guaranteed ways to reduce risk.

Colonoscopies, pap smears, and mammograms help us screen for colon cancer, cervical cancer, and breast cancer, respectively. But there are plenty more types of cancer for which screening is much less commonly performed. Take pancreatic cancer, for example. Pancreatic cancer kills almost as many Americans every year as colon cancer. Similar to how a colonoscopy can help us visualize colon cancer, pancreatic cancer can be seen with CT and MRI scans. Yet, the U.S. Preventive Services Task Force gives pancreatic cancer screening a "D" rating, indicating that the benefits of screening for pancreatic cancer are smaller than the harms.

How can finding cancer earlier not provide a benefit? And how can a screening test cause harm? Pancreatic cancer is known as one of the fastest growing, deadliest cancers around. This means that even if you find it, treatment options may be extremely limited. As such, the U.S. Preventive Services Task Force does not really care if people have their pancreatic cancer detected earlier. They want earlier detection to lead to improved survival. For pancreatic cancer, as well as a whole host of other cancers we do not regularly screen for, early detection does not help people live longer. More people know that they have cancer, but that knowledge does not help treatment.

Plenty of people would prefer not to know that they

have untreatable cancer. For these people, pancreatic cancer screenings would only harm them by forcing them to live under the shadow of a cancer diagnosis. Even commonly performed screening tests have downsides. Anyone who has ever undergone the prep for a colonoscopy knows that sitting on the toilet all night can be rather unpleasant. Mammography turns up plenty of lumps, bumps, and cysts that require patients to undergo further testing. This testing can be scary, painful, and time consuming, and in many cases patients are ultimately told that the mass of concern is completely benign. Taken one way, this is great news. The patient can be relieved that they do not have breast cancer. But the patient also has a right to be angry, having undergone multiple rounds of testing only to be told it was all for nothing, and they would have been just as healthy not having done a mammogram in the first place.

These false positives are why we cannot just screen everyone for every disease. If I scheduled every single patient I saw for a full body MRI scan, I would undoubtedly find a few tumors. It is estimated that about 6% of people have adrenal tumors alone, and pituitary tumors are also quite common. But these tumors are often simply incidental and completely benign, leading doctors to call them 'incidentalomas' when we see them. Still, finding an incidentaloma can trigger a complicated workup.

All those tests come at a cost. Some preventive interventions, specifically childhood vaccines and medical assistance with smoking cessation, can help save money overall by preventing future expenses. But many preventive medicine services, including flu shots, blood pressure checks, and common cancer screenings, are still likely to be a net cost to the healthcare system. That is not necessarily a problem. Spending some money to save lives that would otherwise be lost to preventable illness sounds like a fair tradeoff to me. But preventive medicine, contrary to some popular wisdom, does not necessarily save healthcare dollars.

Decisions about preventive medicine involve weighing complex issues. Every preventive service has benefits. For colonoscopies, the benefit is detecting colon cancer earlier. For flu shots, it is stopping the spread of the flu. But there are also corresponding risks and side effects. Colonoscopy prep essentially forces patients to spend a night on the toilet, and flu shots cause some people to feel feverish or fatigued for a day or so. There is also a financial aspect, both to the healthcare system and to the patient themselves. A patient undergoing a colonoscopy or taking a day off due to feeling achy after a flu shot is not at work making money. For people living paycheck to paycheck, the possibility of missing rent in a week might be much scarier than a potential colon cancer diagnosis years down the line, even if the colonoscopy itself is covered by insurance.

These issues make some preventive services quite controversial, and I would argue no screening test attracts quite as much controversy as screening for prostate cancer. The U.S. Preventive Services Task Force gives prostate cancer screening a "C" rating, indicating the screening should be given based on patient preferences and individual circumstances. The reason for the indecisive recommendation is because the evidence itself is quite mixed. Several large studies examining prostate cancer screening have failed to find that screening prevented prostate cancer deaths. One large study, however, did find that prostate cancer screening lowered the risk of dying from prostate cancer by 20%. On the surface, this sounds like a great result. But a deeper dive into the numbers paints a more complicated picture.

The study found that in the group without prostate cancer screening, five out of every 1,000 men died from prostate cancer during the study's follow up period. In the group that was screened for prostate cancer, four out of every 1,000 men died. That corresponds to a 20% risk reduction, but it means that you would have to screen 1,000 men, quite a crowd, to stop just one prostate cancer death. Since the initial screen for prostate cancer is a simple, low-risk blood test, one could easily argue that it is worth doing as many blood tests as possible.

That being said, the decision gets more complicated. The blood test has a large rate of false positives, and a whopping 17.8% of men screened in the trial ultimately had a false positive result. That means, for every one life saved, 178 men had the stress of a potential cancer scare, without actually having cancer. Of course, these men did not know that their positive screening test was a false positive, so they were advised to undergo a prostate biopsy. While the initial screening test was merely a simple blood draw, a biopsy is a more involved procedure, with about 4% of men developing a fever and 1% requiring hospitalization after their biopsy. In most cases, the biopsy showed that there was no cancer, meaning that the screening provided no benefit to the patient.

Even patients who did receive a prostate cancer diagnosis after their biopsy did not necessarily benefit from the screening. For every 1,000 men who were screened, there were 36 additional prostate cancer diagnoses picked up through screening. But remember, the difference in mortality between the groups was only 1 out of every 1,000. This means that for the vast majority of men with prostate cancer identified through screening, their prostate cancer would not have killed them. Because prostate cancer is often slow growing, men diagnosed with prostate cancer can frequently be treated simply through active monitoring, meaning regular screens to make sure the cancer is not spreading. These men have the benefit of knowing their cancer is being monitored, but also face the mental burden of living with a cancer diagnosis and not receiving any definitive treatment. Many men end up receiving a prostatectomy (the removal of the prostate) to treat the cancer, but these surgeries are associated with an increased risk for urinary incontinence and erectile dysfunction.

Before screening, both patients and doctors should be asking: is it all worth it? Some trials fail to show any benefit from screening. And in the one trial that did show a benefit, every life saved was also associated with other individuals suffering invasive testing, hospitalizations, incontinence, and impotence, all to screen for a cancer that often would not have killed them anyway.

It is not hard to imagine that different people would come to different conclusions on whether prostate cancer screening is "worth it." The patient whose father died of prostate cancer is likely to want the screening. The patient whose father was incontinent for years is likely to fear the potential consequences of a prostate cancer workup. The "C" rating for prostate cancer screening indicates that doctors should have a conversation with patients about the risks and benefits of the screening, and try to make the decision on whether or not to screen together.

The problem here is that prostate cancer screening is just one of many preventive health services. The U.S. Preventive Services Task Force has 46 recommendations receiving either an "A" or "B" rating, suggesting that doctors should offer the service to qualifying patients. Of course, not every recommendation applies to every patient. Women do not need to worry about prostate cancer recommendations, for example. But regardless, doctors have a lot of preventive medicine to discuss at a typical wellness visit. All these discussions, especially if the doctor is trying to do a thorough job of explaining the risks and benefits, take time. When researchers calculated the time it would take a physician to explain and provide all the recommended preventive health services to their patients, they estimated physicians would spend 8.6 hours a day just on preventive health.

Let's assume a typical doctor works from 8AM to 5PM, with a half hour for lunch and a half hour for administrative tasks. That leaves the doctor with eight hours to see patients. With these assumptions, a typical doctor would not have enough time to complete preventive health requirements alone, completely ignoring the sore throats, bad backs, and aching knees that patients want acutely addressed. Time constraints limit the opportunities doctors have to practice the basics of preventive medicine, let alone adequately explain the nuisances of something as complicated as prostate cancer screening.

A typical wellness visit lasts for 20 or 30 minutes. In that time, a doctor is charged with making sure vaccination records are up to date, inquiring about diet and exercise patterns, and discussing a patient's medication list to make sure there are no contraindications and medications are being taken as prescribed. Depending on the patient, the doctor has to think about screening for everything from hypertension and diabetes to HIV and hepatitis, in addition to cancer and depression. Even in a wellness visit, patients might want to talk about their neck pain or problems sleeping. The doctor, meanwhile, might be more concerned about the patient's recent weight gain and lack of exercise. There are so many things to do, and because of time constraints, every item addressed robs time from something else that merits a discussion. No wonder patients are stuck with generic, unhelpful advice like "you really should lose weight" or "you know smoking is bad for you." Patients rightfully should expect more from their doctors, especially about such crucial issues.

How can we fix this? Longer primary care visits would allow more nuanced conversations to occur. But we already have a shortage of primary care doctors, and doctors seeing less patients each day would only further complicate access to primary care. Having nurses or other members of the healthcare team go over medications and offer lifestyle advice would relieve the time burden on doctors, but also complicate the doctor-patient relationship and leave some patients unsatisfied.

Working within the constructs of the current system, I try to start appointments by asking patients what specific things they wish to address during their visit. If the patient has a long list of things to address, I can then suggest deferring wellness discussions to a future visit and focusing on their acute complaints. Patients, of course, can facilitate this prioritization by clearly stating their goals for each visit, even if their doctor does not routinely ask. Doctors and patients together should also be comfortable admitting when things are not working out. If the patient is coming in for a fifth appointment to discuss weight loss, and did not lose any weight after the first four visits, that fifth visit might be a waste of time for both parties.

In fact, some critics of wellness visits will argue that the whole concept is a waste of time. Many components of a stereotypical wellness exam, like listening to the heart and lungs with a stethoscope, palpating lymph nodes, and testing reflexes, are not part of any preventive guidelines at all. In other words, a doctor preforming these exam maneuvers has not been definitely linked to catching disease early or other improvements in health. While an annual physical exam was first recommended by the American Medical Association in the 1920s, most guidelines today focus on screening for specific diseases, and the U.S. Preventive Services Task Force makes no specific recommendation for a comprehensive yearly physical exam in an otherwise healthy adult. In fact, trials evaluating the outcomes of yearly wellness visits have found that they failed to reduce the risks of disability, hospitalization, or death.

In defense of the wellness visit, those trials are far from perfect. Even if a single wellness visit does not magically make people live longer, trials with limited follow up periods are ill-suited to demonstrate the benefit of long-term relationships with a doctor. While wellness visits themselves are not specifically connected with decreased hospitalizations, there is a link between regular outpatient appointments and fewer hospitalizations. Without a designated wellness visit, patients who routinely come in with acute complaints or complex chronic issues might not otherwise have a good opportunity to talk about screening guidelines and preventive medicine with their doctor. A doctor might not want to complicate a visit discussing a new diabetes diagnosis with a depression screen and a discussion about the benefits of a colonoscopy. However, a later wellness visit might pick up the patient's struggle to mentally adapt to their diabetes diagnosis and ensure that the patient is up to date with their cancer screenings. Hospital doctors who face fraught conversations with patient families in the hospital about end-of-life care would find it much easier if primary care doctors had more time to inquire about patient preferences before critical illness. All that being said, perhaps both patients and doctors should acknowledge that testing a healthy 25 year old's reflexes is unlikely to turn up any surprises. Preventive medicine, just like any other facet of healthcare, should be tailored to each individual patient.

The common perception of wellness visits, and preventive medicine in general, is that regular medical checkups help us stop sickness and make diagnoses earlier, letting us better control disease over the long run. The truth is a lot more complicated. The most important aspects of preventive health, maintaining a healthy weight and a high level of physical activity, can be practiced without ever seeing the inside of a doctor's office. And while doctors offer a wide variety of potentially life-saving screenings, any screening comes with potential risks, including false positive findings that lead to complicated workups and treatments. As such, many preventive care strategies actually represent a net cost to both the patient and the health system as a whole, even after factoring in downstream savings. Still, preventive care offers the unique opportunity to stop disease before it even starts, and it is hard to put a price on a trusting, long-term relationship between a patient and their doctor.

CHAPTER 11: GROWING OLD

WHY AGING REQUIRES BOTH LUCK AND SKILL

James Silver makes eye contact with me as I walk in the clinic room, asking, "How's it goin', doc?" through a smile that deepens the joyful wrinkles around his face. Mr. Silver is 70 years old. With white hair, sparkling eyes, and a protuberant belly that he tends to hold with both hands, he reminds me a little bit of Santa. His energy is immediately disarming, but just because he is fun to spend time with does not make him a simple patient to take care of. Weighing 215 pounds on a 5' 10" frame, Mr. Silver's BMI puts him into the obese range. Having been obese for decades, he now faces several comorbidities that were likely caused by his weight. He has high blood pressure, for which he takes a medication called valsartan every morning. He takes a high dose statin medication for elevated cholesterol levels. And five years ago, he was diagnosed with diabetes. The diabetes was first treated with metformin, but he still had issues keeping his sugar levels under control. I recently added a second diabetes medication, semaglutide, and he now seems to be doing much better.

Mr. Silver grumbles about having to take all four medications, but his regimen is nothing special. Around 30 percent of senior citizens regularly take five or more medications, and one study found that 20 percent of individuals aged 70 to 74 were prescribed ten or more medications. In fact, I look at Mr. Silver's blood pressure reading of 140/90 and bring up the possibility of starting a second medication to better control his blood pressure. He waves the idea away, saying that he checks his blood pressure regularly at home and his readings are usually lower.

As much as I would like to discuss the blood pressure issue, Mr. Silver's chief concern today is the worsening pain in his knees. A previous X-ray showed moderate osteoarthritis in both knees, and Mr. Silver says that the pain has started to compromise his mobility. He has already tried topical anti-inflammatory medication, as well as multiple steroid shots. "Doc," he asks, "Am I gonna need a knee replacement?"

Mr. Silver, admittedly, is not a real patient. However, his problems are shared by millions of very real patients all over the county. His most pressing concern, the chronic pain in his knees, is one of those issues that is notoriously difficult to treat. A lot of people expect there to be a magic pill for every complaint. Unfortunately, chronic pain patients are frequently disappointed in the limited options we have to treat them. Exercise is one of the best ways to decrease arthritic knee pain, but performing strengthening activities on an already painful joint can be uncomfortable, especially in people with limited mobility. Moreover, even an intensive diet and exercise plan is unable to dramatically reduce pain for a majority of patients. Anti-inflammatory medications and steroid injections can definitely help control symptoms, but they certainly are not a cure. Chronic pain, often difficult to control even with lifestyle changes and medication, leads many patients like Mr. Silver to consider a surgical option.

Knee replacement surgeries can dramatically improve quality of life, but major surgery carries its own risks. Even patients without surgical complications often face a long recovery process after surgery. Many people are surprised to hear that hip and knee replacements are not perfect fixes, and about 10% of knee replacements need to be revised over a period of twenty years. If Mr. Silver wants to get a knee replacement, he may need to consider the possibility of having yet another surgery down the road.

What Mr. Silver is facing, both with his knee pain and his medical conditions, are the accumulated comorbidities from decades of being overweight and inactive. Once developed, many of these conditions, like arthritis, hypertension and diabetes, become chronic. Mr. Silver might be unhappy with the limited treatment options for his knee pain, but for his other conditions, medical advances have greatly improved his quality of life. In "The Boscombe Valley Mystery" by Sir Author Conan Doyle, Sherlock Holmes' accomplice Dr. Watson sees a man with longstanding diabetes and remarks, "It was clear to me at a glance that he was in the grip of some deadly and chronic disease." Medicine has greatly improved since Dr. Watson's observation was published in 1891, and doctors today should not be able to diagnose well-managed diabetes on sight. Mr. Silver, also with longstanding diabetes, can at least sleep well-assured that his diabetes is controlled and unlikely to kill him.

Just by taking his medications and keeping his blood sugars in check, Mr. Silver should be able to escape many complications of his diabetes diagnosis.

But while modern medicine has become very good at controlling some chronic diseases, Mr. Silver still would have been better off having implemented diet and lifestyle changes years ago. These changes could have prevented him from developing the diabetes, high cholesterol, and high blood pressure he now wishes he did not have to take medications to control. The good news is that Mr. Silver can still make meaningful changes to improve his well-being now. Many studies have shown that improved diet and exercise, even in middle and older age, can greatly benefit health and quality of life. Modern medicine can even help spur these changes along. Mr. Silver's semaglutide, prescribed as a diabetes treatment, has a side effect of considerable weight loss. If Mr. Silver loses ten pounds from being on semaglutide, the extra weight off his aching knees might help him increase his physical activity. A century ago, Mr. Silver would have had even fewer options to treat his knee pain, likely leading to less and less mobility over time. Since physical activity is such an important component of managing his chronic diseases, being wheelchair bound would be devastating for his health. A knee replacement surgery, thanks to the wonders of modern medicine, might help keep him active for decades to come.

The lessons from Mr. Silver's case are clear. Lifestyle decisions in our younger years do eventually add up over time, often leading to comorbidities later in life. While modern medicine can manage chronic disease, it is of course better to not develop the disease in the first place. While some treatments, like Mr. Silver's medications, are effective with minimal side effects, other interventions, like the knee replacement he is considering, are much more invasive. Medicine has come a long way, but it is still better to not need it in the first place.

Unfortunately, managing chronic disease is a key part of life for almost anyone navigating the aging process. Sooner or later, pretty much everyone develops some health issue that requires medical management. Good management of our conditions can help them fade into the background with minimal effects on health. Poor management can lead to complications and decreased quality of life. Some treatments, like undergoing a knee replacement surgery for an arthritic joint, are essentially cures. But for a lot of conditions, all we can really do is try to reduce the risk of complications.

To demonstrate this point, let me introduce you to another hypothetical patient, Emilia Gold. Ms. Gold is a 81 year old retired widow. She lives alone, and is fiercely proud of her independence. For her age, Ms. Gold is a shockingly healthy lady. She was treated for breast cancer 15 years ago, but has had no recurrence since then. Her only chronic condition is her high blood pressure. Various doctors have tried to treat her with a succession of high blood pressure pills, but she complains about the side effects of each one. Chlorthalidone made her wake up to pee, amlodipine made her feet swell, and lisinopril gave her a mild cough. She is now technically prescribed losartan, but when I ask her if she is actually taking it, she replies, "Some of the time." When pressed to offer specifics about how frequently that means, she sidesteps the question. I would be surprised if she were taking the medication at all.

Even more frustrating than Ms. Gold's resistance to her high blood pressure medication is her smoking habit. She only smokes about a half a pack of cigarettes a day, she reminds me, ignoring the fact that over 60 years of her smoking, her habit has added up to over 200,000 cigarettes. It might seem shocking that

Ms. Gold has lived to 81 as a smoker without developing lung cancer. But believe it or not, she actually has the odds on her side. Although around 90% of lung cancers occur in smokers, only 15% percent of smokers eventually contract lung cancer. Similarly, high blood pressure certainly raises the risk for heart attacks and strokes, but just having high blood pressure does not automatically mean someone is bound to develop these complications.

Ms. Gold serves as a reminder that aging is all about managing risks. She could have decreased her lifetime risk of lung cancer by not smoking in the first place, or even by quitting long ago. But while many people with her smoking history do develop and frequently die of lung cancer, others are able to live into their eighties happily smoking away. In a way, the constant risks we face as we grow old make aging something like walking through a minefield. We can take every precaution and plan our route well, but our ultimate fate is beyond is our control. Some people, through sheer bad luck, face devastating diagnoses well before they reach old age. Other individuals, including Ms. Gold, can accumulate multiple risk factors and walk away unscarred.

The majority of what we perceive as healthy habits, including everything from eating well and being active to wearing our seatbelt and taking medications as prescribed, is us trying to minimize our risk factors. Still, it is impossible to completely eliminate every risk. At the end of the day, a fit, healthy 40 year old can die in a car accident or from an unexpected cancer, and their next door neighbor can turn 100 in spite of multiple comorbidities.

As scary as this may sound, medicine has done a great job of stacking the odds in our favor. Mr. Silver can expect to live many more years in spite of his multiple comorbidities. A century ago, this would not have been the case. And Ms. Gold is already a cancer survivor, having been in remission from breast cancer for over a decade. Caught early through a routine mammogram, Ms. Gold's cancer was treated before it had the chance to spread beyond her breast. The five year survival rate for localized breast cancer, due to early diagnosis and excellent treatment options, is a stunning 99 percent. Smoking cigarettes likely increased the risk of Ms. Gold developing breast cancer. But thanks to modern medicine, Ms. Gold's breast cancer diagnosis was simply a minor blip in an otherwise healthy life.

Doctors treating an acute issue, like oncologists giving chemotherapy for cancer or hospital doctors giving antibiotics for pneumonia, can offer patients the promise of a definitive cure. But much of modern medicine is treating chronic diseases, where no cure is possible. Doctors cannot promise Mr. Silver that his statin will stop him from having a heart attack, or that his valsartan will stop him from having a stroke. Instead, these medications are designed to lower his risk, increasing his odds of continued good health.

But even as medicine has become better and better at treating both acute and chronic disease, most people would prefer not taking all of Mr. Silver's medications or having Ms. Gold's breast cancer scare. Medicine is great, but not needing it is even better. So, what can we do to give ourselves the best chance at aging well?

Many studies have tried to address this question, but the most famous is certainly the Harvard Study of Adult Development. Starting during the Great Depression, Harvard tracked cohorts of its students, giving them routine surveys on health and wellbeing, as well as asking about their lifestyles. The study can be easily criticized for its unrepresentative sample, as the almost uniformly wealthy, white men studying at Harvard (when the study began, women were not yet allowed entry as Harvard undergraduates) hardly embodied all of America. To give an idea of just how privileged the sample was, future president John F. Kennedy was included in one of the original cohorts. However, the study later expanded to include a more representative population, and by longitudinally tracking the same participants for over seven decades, the Study of Adult Development gives us unparalleled data on the aging process.

Results from the study show that some aspects of aging are simply beyond our control. Ancestral longevity, years of education received, and physical health at age 50 all helped predict participants' health and wellbeing as they aged. In other words, it can be hard to escape our genes and our upbringing. Thankfully, other predictors of healthy aging were more controllable, including regular exercise, a normal BMI, and limited alcohol consumption. These findings, also backed up by the countless studies already discussed throughout this book, are hardly surprising. But notably, the Study of Adult Development found that a stable marriage and mature defense mechanisms helped improve both mental and physical health as subjects aged. For as much as we discuss healthy eating and physical activity as the cornerstones of healthy aging, the Study of Adult Development tells us that healthy, stable relationships are just as important. For all the risks associated with the aging process, the study offers a promising conclusion: "One may have greater personal control over... health after retirement than previously recognized."

The Study of Adult Development is not the only study indicating that there is more to growing old than just good genes, physical activity, and healthy eating. One study found that elderly subjects who engaged in mentally stimulating leisure activities such as reading, competing in board games, and playing musical instruments were less likely to develop dementia than their peers who had less cognitive stimulation. Another trial used a high-quality, randomized-controlled design to test the effect of cognitive training in elderly participants, finding that older subjects could be trained to have better memory, reasoning, and speed. Impressively, these improvements were maintained after five years of follow-up, demonstrating longitudinal benefits of keeping one's mind active.

Strong engagement with family, friends, and the wider community also seems to have noticeable benefits on aging. Multiple studies have shown that individuals with a higher quantity and quality of social relationships tend to have longer life expectancies. Importantly, even individuals who otherwise lack many strong relationships seem to benefit from new social connections. One study followed elderly individuals given volunteer roles in nearby elementary schools, providing them with mentally stimulating tasks as well as new relationships. After just a few months of volunteering, subjects noted improvements in social connections, cognitive ability, physical activity, and strength.

The fact that elderly volunteers saw improvements in both mental and physical health underscores the close dynamic between the two. Skeptics questioning the results from the Study of Adult Development can find fault with the study's focus on strong relationships and coping strategies. Their argument is fairly simple: loneliness does not kill people; heart attacks, strokes, and cancer do. Even scientists discussing aging studies note that it can be incredibly difficult to determine which behaviors ultimately lead to poor health. Few people would disagree that heavy alcohol use can cause negative health effects, and the Study of Adult Development offers concrete data supporting that argument. But researchers trying to determine if loneliness leads to increased alcohol use or heavy alcohol use leads to social isolation can give themselves a headache trying to figure out which causes which. Are people with stable relationships able to be healthier because they have companions to keep them active? Or are inactive people simply less able to go out and meet new people?

These sorts of questions become classic 'chicken or the egg' issues, where it is hard if not impossible to tell which risk factor came first. In general, it is fair to say that biological, psychological, and social aspects of health are all intertwined. If one is biologically unwell, say bedbound and unable to care for themselves, their mental and social health are likely to suffer. Someone suffering from a psychological issue, say depression, is less likely to be physically active and be able to maintain strong social ties. And someone who is socially isolated has less reasons to leave the house and may psychologically suffer as well. Research increasingly invokes a 'biopsychosocial' model of health, incorporating all the various biological, psychological, and social components.

The biopsychosocial model captures a broader picture of our overall health and wellbeing than the more traditional medical model, which focuses on specific disease states like diabetes or hypertension. Enlarging our definition of health helps us be more creative in our treatments. Sure, diabetes and hypertension can be countered with medication, which helps treat the biological underpinnings of each disease. But the biopsychosocial model views both diseases as consequences of limited activity and poor diet, giving us broader treatment options. A healthy eating group meeting once weekly could help Mr. Silver find recipes to improve his diet, as well as the social support he may need to maintain healthy changes. A new friend he meets at that group might encourage him to join his regular golf outing, helping him improve his level of physical activity. If Ms. Gold joined a senior citizen club, positive peer pressure might finally convince her to stop smoking or take her medication.

Healthy aging is complex. Not only must we acknowledge that we do not have complete control over our health as we age, but we must also acknowledge that risk factors develop from every aspect of our lives: biological, psychological, and social. Fortunately, our healthy habits can also flourish from these same domains, diversifying our ways of managing risk. There is no one trick to a long, healthy life. To age well, we need good health, a strong mind, and meaningful relationships. We also need quite a bit of luck.

CHAPTER 12: DEATH

WHY THAT ICE CREAM IS PROBABLY WORTH IT

Plenty of high-quality scientific studies offer strong evidence on how to live a longer life. The Mediterranean diet can increase life expectancy. Having a healthy BMI decreases the risk of mortality. The right medications help reduce the possibility of potentially deadly events like heart attacks and strokes. All of these outcomes are fantastic, but they obscure an unwelcome truth. No matter how many vegetables we eat, how proud we are of our waistlines, or how many medications we can swallow, we all eventually die.

We often delude ourselves into thinking we have a lot more control over death than we actually do. Not only can it be existentially uncomfortable to ponder our own mortality, but media also gives us an inaccurate picture of how effective medicine can be. In movies and television, the hospital staff only has to push lightly on the patient's chest during cardiopulmonary resuscitation (CPR) to miraculously bring them back to life. In real life, CPR breaks bones. For all of modern medicine's fancy technology and impressive gadgetry, CPR might be the most primitive thing we do – repeatedly compressing a patient's chest in the hope of squeezing some blood out of a malfunctioning heart. CPR is so physical that most people, even trained professionals, struggle to maintain high quality chest compressions for more than two minutes. And for all that effort, the vast majority of patients requiring CPR never leave the hospital alive. Of course, you would not know that shocking statistic just from watching TV. Patients who receive CPR on television are two times as likely to regain a heartbeat as they are in real life. They are up to four times more likely to survive to hospital discharge.

Just like pharmacology or physiology, death is a part of training for doctors. My very first class of medical school was anatomy, complete with cadaver dissection. For obvious reasons, the last names of the cadavers were hidden, but the anatomy professors purposefully shared their first names. The lesson was straightforward. These were not just bodies; they were people. The very first patient I admitted to the hospital as a medical student never left alive. Time and time again, I have seen the slow realization dawn in the eyes of a patient's family as they began to understand that their loved one would not get any better.

Doctors spend a solid portion of their lives among the dead and dying. And yet the average patient is unaccustomed to contemplating death. This discord can be problematic when doctors and patients need to work together to decide on the goals of a patient's care. Every single patient admitted to the hospital needs to be asked about their code status, a term doctors use to determine if a patient wants to receive CPR and mechanical ventilation if their heart and lungs were to fail. Doctors have different ways of asking this question. I generally ask, "If for some reason your heart were to stop, or you couldn't breathe on your own, would you want us to do CPR and place a breathing tube down your throat?"

Some patients have a yes or no answer, but I also receive a lot of answers along the lines of "It depends.", "Can I think about it?", and "I don't know." Noncommittal answers generally result in the doctor marking the patient down as a full code, meaning the hospital would do everything in its power to keep the patient alive. But when given more time to think things through, or when hearing the code status question phrased differently, patients often change their minds. One study found that patient preferences for their code status differed from what doctors had entered into their chart a staggering 20% of the time. Such a high error rate is deeply disturbing when code status discussions are truly a matter of life or death.

Doctors complain about receiving unclear code status preferences all the time. But should medical experts really be surprised when less informed individuals want more knowledge before making such a tremendous decision? Likely affected by media portrayals of CPR, patients tend to overestimate the effectiveness of resuscitation methods. When given more information on CPR's effectiveness, many change their minds. Outside of TV and movies, only about 10% of patients who experience a cardiac arrest outside of the hospital will be alive one month later. Sure, CPR success rates are higher in the hospital, but this good news is countered by the fact that simply surviving a cardiac arrest does not necessarily mean a return to one's previous level of health. Many cardiac arrest survivors experience debilitating neurological trauma.

All of this information does not mean that CPR is worthless. On the contrary, it saves lives every day, and I firmly believe that everyone should know the basics to potentially become a literal lifesaver. But I also believe that society's unrealistic view of CPR outcomes is emblematic of a larger, overly optimistic view we have toward death. Healthy diets and intense exercise regimens are billed at stopping the aging process, but even vegan ultramarathon runners eventually grow old. We may not want to die, but we all have to prepare for it.

Admittedly, we do have some good reasons for optimism about the aging process. Over the years from 1840 to 2000, life expectancy for the healthiest individuals in wealthy nations increased from about 45 years to 85 years. That corresponds to almost a doubling of life expectancy. Even more amazingly, maternal death rates have fallen about 99% since the dawn of the industrial revolution. Similarly, infant death rates have plummeted. A family losing a few young children to untimely deaths used to be the norm. Now, new parents expect their children to reach adulthood safely.

More exciting news may be on the horizon. In one study, scientists discovered that patients with diabetes who were taking the common diabetes medication metformin lived longer on average than patients without diabetes. At first glance, these results are confusing. Diabetes is a chronic disease associated with an increased risk of heart attacks and infections. Why then were people with diabetes living longer than people without it?

The answer, scientists concluded, might have something to do with the metformin. Animal studies have found that regular doses of metformin increase the average lifespan of mice and roundworms. In humans, metformin is associated with a decreased risk of cancer. Since metformin has been around for decades and is used by millions of people with diabetes, we know it is generally safe. And in stark opposition to many newer drugs that cost thousands of dollars, metformin is sold for just a few dollars a month. If doctors wanted to repurpose a drug to fight aging, metformin seems like the ideal candidate.

There is, undoubtedly, some good evidence in favor of metformin as an anti-aging drug. But there are two sides to every story. Metformin use does have some side effects, most commonly nausea and diarrhea. People taking metformin are also at increased risk for developing scary complications like vitamin B12 deficiency and lactic acidosis. Yet again, we learn that no drug is perfect. And even though metformin has had promising effects on extending the lifespan of roundworms and mice, it has had no effect on lifespan for rats and fruit flies. Metformin research remains promising, but a simple medication is unlikely to be a cure for the aging process.

Like metformin, caloric restriction has recently been touted as an anti-aging therapy. Caloric restriction is the concept of eating up to 50% less calories than a usual diet. In numerous animal studies, caloric restriction extends lifespan. But applying this logic to humans is fraught with complications. Unlike mice in cages, us humans have complex mental and physical tasks requiring our energy every day. We cannot simply sit around lethargic and famished, even if it might help us live longer. Laboratory mice are often used in experiments because they live similar, unexciting lives. Humans, on the other hand, face more variable medical needs. Recommending that an obese 40 year old cut calories makes a lot of sense. Recommending the same to a frail 80 year old is likely ill advised.

Just as importantly, people like to eat. Unlike laboratory mice, humans have control over their own food, and many people reasonably would not want to go through life always feeling hungry. Caloric restriction proponents argue that we can simply develop drugs that copy caloric restriction's biochemical effects. But for the time being, these anti-aging drugs are more science fiction than actual science.

In fact, even as medicine and public health have worked together to dramatically increase the average human lifespan over the last 200 years, we have done astonishingly little to increase the maximum lifespan. Eighty and ninety year-old people are far from a new phenomenon. Many of America's founding fathers, including Thomas Jefferson and Benjamin Franklin, lived well into their eighties. John Adams survived into his nineties. Living to old age is certainly much more common today, but the definition of old age itself has hardly shifted. U.S. life expectancy has roughly doubled since the time of America's founding. But while Benjamin Franklin could serve in the Continental Congress at age 81 back in 1787, there are not any 162 year-old politicians today.

Might we make progress on extending lifespan in the future? Is aging, just like pneumonia or diabetes, something that can be treated medically? Perhaps, but there is certainly no guarantee right now. Medical science is advancing at an unforeseen pace, offering great hope for future breakthroughs. At the same time, scientists have been searching for a way to extend lifespan for centuries, and yet people still grow old and die.

For the time being, all we can do is try to live a healthy life. But the knowledge that we cannot cheat illness and death, only avoid them temporarily, complicates our decisions. The person who eats an immaculate diet without a gram of added sugar will still eventually age and die. So too will the person who wakes up every morning for a five mile run. Statistically, health-conscious individuals will live longer on average than people who make less healthy decisions. But averages become less important when we only have one life to live. Sure, a healthy diet can lower the risk of diabetes, hypertension, and even cancer. But lifestyle alone cannot completely eliminate the risk of any of these diseases.

Quality lifestyle choices offer us better odds of good health and long life, but they also force us to make some sacrifices. Maintaining a healthy diet means that we cannot eat multiple servings of our favorite dessert each night. It also requires the economic flexibility to buy nutritious options that are often more expensive. Exercise and sleep regimens take time out of our already busy lives, and can limit the time we spend with our loved ones. While doctors rightly recommend a healthy lifestyle as protection against a staggering array of diseases, we would be mistaken to ignore the fact that lifestyle changes often put significant burdens on our patients.

People approach the tradeoff between the diligence required to maintain a healthy lifestyle and the benefits such a lifestyle provides in different ways. Some people make considerable sacrifices to treat their body as well as possible, abstaining from unhealthy foods and spending many hours a week on exercise. Others choose to eat whatever they want, whenever they want, and live a largely sedentary lifestyle.

As a doctor, I have worked with patients in both camps, but also believe that we can all find some middle ground. People who enjoy extensive physical activity and carefully controlling their diet of course reap the rewards of these healthy lifestyle choices. But the rest of us can still make big strides toward improving our health with slightly less strict regimens.

I will offer my own lifestyle as an example of this middle ground approach. I try my best to stay physically active, frequently taking time to go on neighborhood walks or bike rides. On a rare day off, I might chart out a four or five mile hike in a local natural area. When buying groceries, I make a concerted effort to plan healthy meals, and have made plant-forward, Mediterranean style dishes weekly staples.

On the flip side, my motivation to lift weights admittedly waxes and wanes, meaning that I do not always meet the two days a week of strength training recommended in the Physical Activity Guidelines for Americans. And as much as I try to buy healthy foods, I have a particular weakness for ice cream. Medicine is hard, and daydreaming about a dessert at the end of the day helps keep my mood up. Is ice cream healthy? No, but against the background of an otherwise fairly healthy lifestyle, I view it as an acceptable luxury. Life is short, and I certainly do not want to make it any shorter with poor lifestyle choices. But there is also no reason for me to use my time trying to avoid every possible risk factor. So for the time being, I will continue to enjoy the occasional hefty scoop of ice cream.

In fact, doctors are not always completely sure about the health effects of specific lifestyle choices. Take, for example, occasional alcohol use. Heavy drinking has well known health risks, but some studies show that people who report light alcohol use, say one glass of wine a few days a week, live longer than people who abstain completely from alcohol. However, opposing studies note that many people who abstain from alcohol do so due to poor health or a history of heavy alcohol use. These people, sicker on average than the general population, may skew the results. The exact conclusions differ from study to study, meaning that despite years of targeted research, there is no clear answer on the exact health effects of occasional drinking. In general, previous claims that occasional drinking has health benefits have started to shift toward skepticism of any alcohol intake, with the World Health Organization declaring in 2023 that no level of alcohol consumption is safe.

Doctors do not have a ready answer for every question. Some questions, like "Is heavy drinking bad for you?" are easily answered by decades of data. But other questions, including "Is my daily glass of red wine good or bad for me?" are difficult to answer. And ironically, especially for a profession whose training pathway exposes us to the dead and dying, doctors have no good answer for one of the most important questions of all, "What happens after death?"

Since doctors come from all faiths and creeds, there is certainly no medical answer to such a question. Both popular news and scientific studies share reports of cardiac arrest survivors describing bright lights, mystical beings, and intense feelings of joy and peace during the time that they were pulseless. Many of these reports also include an out-of-body experience, where the survivor saw their own body lying in the hospital bed from above. Those who are religiously inclined can point to these experiences as evidence for continued existence after death. More agnostic observers argue that these experiences can be explained as simple hallucinations from a dying brain.

Testing whether or not these otherworldly descriptions are actually supernatural phenomena or mere sensory illusions seems like a task beyond the scope of science. However, one team of researchers developed an ingenious study protocol to put these near-death experiences to the test. Hearing many reports of cardiac arrest survivors describing experiences where they floated above their body, these researchers placed random images on hospital shelves that would only be visible to the patient if their consciousness actually rose above their body during cardiac resuscitation. Imagine, for example, a cardiac arrest survivor noticing an American flag and a picture of a giraffe high on a hospital shelf only visible to a presence floating many feet over their hospital bed. As incredible as it sounds, these researchers had concocted a study to provide scientific evidence of consciousness after death.

These researchers, titling their study AWARE (short for AWAreness during REsuscitation), placed hundreds of images across 15 hospitals, then planned to interview willing cardiac arrest survivors to record how they described their own cardiac arrest. In the participating hospitals, 2060 cardiac arrests were noted, with 330 cardiac arrest survivors. Of these survivors, 140 were willing and able to give interviews. Many described feelings of peace, heightened senses, or separation from their bodies. However, only one was able to give an accurate representation of events that occurred during his cardiac arrest, saying that he perceived his own resuscitation from a vantage point outside his body in the top corner of the room.

This story matched perfectly with the out-of-body experience the researchers had planned for. But the hospital room in which this cardiac arrest occurred did not have any images installed on its shelf. As such, the AWARE team were unable to confirm the story. In a study encompassing over 2000 cardiac arrests, not a single surviving patient was able to identify any of the images placed by the researchers.

While it would be nice to know what comes after death, the difficulties encountered by the AWARE researchers demonstrate that any scientific proof may be hard to come by. And even if the AWARE study had found a survivor who claimed to see an image left on a shelf by researchers, both skeptics and religious individuals would be quick to argue over how the results should be interpreted.

Without any proof of what comes next, we should all feel entitled to choose our beliefs and live our lives with as much meaning as possible. Much of medicine is about trying to stave off death, even as we are totally in the dark about what comes after. But just as we all are free to have our own opinions on death, we are also free to choose our own tradeoffs between healthy choices and guilty pleasures. Even as death remains an enigma, I ask patients to consider their attitudes toward their eventual demise, and I encourage everyone to communicate their code status preference with loved ones. If we only get one life, we should all be aware of exactly how we want to live it, but also how we want it to end.

CHAPTER 13: FINAL THOUGHTS

WHY DOCTORS AND PATIENTS CAN'T GIVE UP ON EACH OTHER

Most formal K-12 schooling includes the basics of math, history, and English. But even as most of us forget the complexities of algebra, the War of 1812, and transcendentalist writers, we face diagnoses and health challenges that force us to interact with the healthcare system. And for how crucial it is to maintain health over the course of our lives, most people learn very little medicine.

Admittedly, the average patient does not need to know the precise mechanism of action, contraindications, and specific pharmacologic interactions of their blood pressure medication. That sort of knowledge should largely be the responsibility of the doctor prescribing it. And yet, I would argue that we should all, doctors and patients alike, know both the risks of high blood pressure itself, and also how to lower it. After all, nearly half of American adults have high blood pressure, and millions of Americans are taking prescription medication for this condition. That being said, prescription medications are far from the only way to control one's blood pressure. Comprehensive dietary changes can spur a ten point drop of blood pressure on average. Overweight individuals who lose ten pounds can expect to see about a five point drop in their blood pressure. Cutting salt intake, even in the absence of any weight loss, can have a similar effect. This is important and possibly lifesaving information, but is not included in a typical high school or even college curriculum. By frequently constricting medical education to people pursuing medicine as a career, our society limits access to information that might otherwise empower individuals to take better control over their own health.

As a result, many people enter medical interactions knowing little about the conditions they face. In turn, patients are forced to place a great deal of trust in their doctors, hoping they are receiving accurate information without being subjected to unnecessary testing and expensive treatments. Doctors, knowing the medical rationale behind their patient care decisions, often forget to put themselves in their patients' shoes. This oversight is not just poor bedside manner. It can also be dangerous, as mistrust and misunderstandings put patient lives at risk.

Picture a patient with some skepticism about the medical field going to their first wellness visit in many years. There, a doctor they have never met before informs them that they have hypertension, and they are handed a prescription for hydrochlorothiazide, a medication they are told will lower their blood pressure. The doctor gets to walk away from this visit feeling satisfied, confident they have successfully helped manage the patient's blood pressure, lowering the risk of future heart attacks and strokes.

But unfortunately for the doctor's ego, just writing a prescription does not improve health outcomes. High blood pressure often has no physical symptoms, so the patient can easily conclude that their hypertension is not a big issue, deciding not to take the prescribed pills. They might show up at the pharmacy intending to fill the prescription, only to be dismayed by the cost and decide the medication is not worth it. Even after buying the medication, they can decide they are unhappy with the side effect of increased urinary frequency, leaving the rest of the pills unused on some bathroom shelf. Or they can even return to the doctor confidently proclaiming they are taking their medication as prescribed, when in fact they misunderstood the exact dosing and frequency.

These sorts of barriers to proper medication use are frighteningly common. An estimated 20 to 30% of prescriptions written each year are never filled, and an estimated 50% of medications for chronic diseases like high blood pressure and diabetes are not taken as prescribed. Doctors call this phenomenon medication nonadherence, and it is estimated to be responsible for 10% of all hospital admissions, causing 125,000 American deaths a year. By naming the problem medication nonadherence, doctors conveniently place the blame on their patients for not taking their medications as prescribed. However, physician reminders, additional patient education, and shared decision making all help increase patient compliance with medications, showing that doctors still have plenty of tools to work with. Treating a patient's condition simply cannot stop with a doctor writing a prescription and hoping for the best.

All these issues with medication noncompliance can

occur even if a patient likes and trusts their doctor. But there are plenty of people who have deep distrust of the healthcare system. One poll found that 36% of respondents agreed with the statement "Medical experiments can be done on me without me knowing about it." 58% of respondents agreed that "If a mistake were made in my health care, the health care system would try to hide it from me." 71% agreed that "Some medicines have things in them that they do not tell you about."

This depth of skepticism, I would argue, is a little unfair. But it is hardly unexpected, especially considering frequent reports of fraudulent medical billing, sexism and racism from healthcare professionals, and even criminal charges against physicians. Even us doctors who try to follow the rules cannot seem to agree with each other. One study examined patients referred to the Mayo Clinic for a second opinion, finding that in 21% of referrals, the second opinion resulted in a "distinctly different" diagnosis. An incorrect diagnosis can be catastrophic, and certainly should not be commonplace. All in all, there are plenty of reasons patients have to doubt the advice of their doctors. Unfortunately, this distrust of the healthcare system has consequences, and individuals with less trust in healthcare institutions tend to delay potentially lifesaving care.

Not everything is bad news. I can personally attest that the vast majority of healthcare workers I have encountered in my career are kind, dedicated, and focused on doing the best for their patients. And some of the reports decrying deeply rooted issues within the healthcare system may be overstating their case. Many healthcare skeptics claim that medical error is the third most frequent cause of death in the United States. These claims largely trace back to a 2016 article in the British Medical Journal calculating that medical errors led to a shocking 251,000 deaths just in the U.S. each year. But while the article's conclusion became widely cited as a fact, the research design itself has been met with intense criticism. For example, the article assumed that any patient death occurring after any medical error was automatically caused by the error. So if a patient received an antibiotic to which they had a previously documented allergy, then developed a minor rash, the erroneously prescribed antibiotic would be counted as killing the patient, even if the patient died of a completely unrelated cause many days later. Other research, although less frequently cited, finds the rate of preventable deaths due to medical error occurring at less than 10% of the rate claimed by the British Medical Journal article.

Patients often complain that they feel rushed and ignored by their doctors. But the issue is not just as simple as doctors lacking empathy. Facing long days of complex cognitive and emotional tasks, as well as cramped patient schedules often imposed by nonclinical administrators, many doctors are just doing their best to tread water. At the same time, with lawsuits being commonplace, many doctors are forced to practice medicine worrying more about being sued than the welfare of the patient in front of them. Documentation requirements have increased dramatically in recent years, both to protect against lawsuits and to store information in electronic health records. Many doctors now spend more time with computers than patients, with a recent study estimating that physicians average over 16 minutes on the computer for each patient visit.

The result? American doctors face burnout at record rates, with many studies showing a majority of U.S. physicians reporting symptoms of burnout. Scarily, these symptoms are often associated with adverse effects on both patient and physician health. At the same time, large swaths of the country have deep distrust of doctors and the medical system at a whole, often delaying or preventing skeptics from seeking needed care.

The American healthcare system has somehow transformed into an unwieldly mess alienating both doctors and their patients.

What can we do? Let's diagnose the problem before we try to treat it. There are a whole host of issues with healthcare in the United States. But patients expressing distrust towards their doctors and doctors feeling burnt out by patient care are two symptoms of the same underlying problem: a weakening of the doctor-patient relationship. A couple of generations ago, patients enjoyed longitudinal relationships with their community physician, looking to their doctor as their main source of medical information. Now, decades of mergers and the rise of corporate medicine have led many doctors to practice as part of large physician groups, and changing insurance rules mean that patients often have to find a new doctor. Patients are exposed to large quantities of medical information on the TV and internet, with many sources being of dubious quality at best. And by being employees of larger networks, as well as by having to juggle patient care with copious documentation requirements, doctors are often limited in the amount of time they can spend with each patient.

Even as we complain about the current system, doctors and our professional organizations hold great sway over how healthcare is organized and delivered. As such, physician groups should advocate for programs that help dismantle barriers our patients face in both accessing and affording healthcare. Clinics and hospitals should foster inclusive environments so that patients do not feel like their care is affected by their race, gender, or income level. Individual doctors should always look beyond their patients' medical diagnoses to consider the social, economic, and psychological factors affecting health. Prescribing a medication a patient cannot afford or will not ultimately take is no better than failing to prescribe a medication at all. By sharing decisions with patients about the different options available to them, doctors can foster a sense of partnership that increases patient confidence in their treatment plan. And although it may hurt our egos, recommending second opinions when patients face complex decisions allows our patients to be more comfortable with their final diagnoses.

But since doctors face hectic schedules and competing demands, we should also invite patients to actively participate in their own care. National health organizations, like the American Heart Association and the American Lung Association, put out lots of quality online content directed at educating patients. Doctors can also direct patients to high-quality government sources, including the CDC website and Medline Plus, from the National Library of Medicine. Patients can help their doctors by sending information from outside health systems to their doctor's office in advance of their appointment. New patients who come with their medication list ready, and returning patients who come with a list of questions, also help ensure that their appointments go smoothly. If an elderly relative has a doctor's appointment, family should find someone to accompany them and then double check they are taking their medications as prescribed. Too many elderly patients, just like our friend Ms. Gold, show up to all their doctors' appointments only to concoct their own medication regimens as soon as they get home. And while you should never let a doctor rush your appointment, please understand that if we are running behind schedule it is probably because we were busy with another patient, not relaxing in the breakroom.

The landscape of American medicine has drastically changed in recent decades. While new scientific and technological innovations have helped the lives of many, increasing costs and decreasing access to care have angered both doctors and patients alike. No single reform will be sufficient to fix every flaw in our current system. But I still believe that the core of medicine lies in the doctor-patient relationship, and that both doctors and patients can make simple strides towards strengthening this relationship for the modern era. Modern life, just like the practice of medicine, is at once complex, beautiful, terrifying, and exhausting. We could all do better by treating everyone we meet with an extra dose of kindness.

REFERENCES

<u>Chapter 1</u>

"locals boast that they frequently live to age 100" Mazess, R.B. Health and longevity in Vilcabamba, Ecuador. JAMA. 1978; 240(16): 1781.

"elderly locals were able to show" Sullivan, Walter. Very old people in the Andes are found to be merely old. New York Times. 1978, Mar 17, pg. A8.

"locals frequently exaggerated their ages" Mazess, R.B. & Forman, S.H. Longevity and age exaggeration in Vilcabamba, Ecuador. Journal of Gerontology. 1979; 34(1): 94-98.

"the proportion of elderly villagers" Mazess, R.B. & Mathisen, R.W. Lack of unusual longevity in Vilcabamba, Ecuador. Human Biology. 1982; 54(3): 517-524.

"The American Dental Association recommends" Flossing. MouthHealthy.org. American Dental Association.

https://www.mouthhealthy.org/en/az-topics/f/flossing/
"flossing can reduce levels of gum inflammation" Sälzer S, Slot DE, Van der Weijden FA, Dörfer CE. Efficacy of inter-dental mechanical plaque control in managing gingivitis--a meta-review. J Clin Periodontol. 2015 Apr;42 Suppl 16:S92-105.
"That being said, some researchers question" Berchier CE, Slot DE, Haps S, Van der Weijden GA. The efficacy of dental floss in addition to a toothbrush on plaque and parameters of gingival inflammation: a systematic review. Int J Dent Hyg. 2008 Nov;6(4):265-79.
"the mere act of flossing" Church, Chocolate, Sex and 3 Other Keys to Living Longer. http://www.cbsnews.com/8301-505146_162-39943623/church-chocolate-sex-and-3-other-keys-to-living-longer/
"a 1999 book called RealAge" Roizen M. RealAge: Are You as Young as You Could Be? Diane Publishing Company; 1999
"a 1993 study" DeStefano F, Anda RF, Kahn HS, et al. Dental disease and risk of coronary heart disease and mortality. BMJ. 1993 Mar 13;306(6879):688-91.
"less likely to be overweight" Hujoel PP, Cunha-Cruz J, Kressin NR. Spurious associations in oral epidemiological research: the case of dental flossing and obesity. Journal of Clinical Periodontology. 2006;33(8):520-523.
"as study after study" Sacks FM, Pfeffer MA, Moye LA, et al. The Effect of Pravastatin on Coronary Events after Myocardial Infarction in Patients with Average Cholesterol Levels. New England Journal of Medicine. 1996;335(14):1001-1009.
"can reduce deaths from heart attacks and strokes" LaRosa JC, Grundy SM, Waters DD, et al. Intensive Lipid Lowering with Atorvastatin in Patients with Stable Coronary Disease. New England Journal of Medicine. 2005;352(14):1425-1435.
"most common side effect" Rosenson RS, Baker S, Banach M,

et al. Optimizing Cholesterol Treatment in Patients With
Muscle Complaints. J Am Coll Cardiol. 2017;70(10):1290-1301.

"doctors generally respond to these side effects" Toth PP, Patti
AM, Giglio RV, et al. Management of Statin Intolerance in
2018: Still More Questions Than Answers. Am J Cardiovasc
Drugs. 2018;18(3):157-173.

"taking Coenzyme Q10 can help" Qu H, Guo M, Chai H,
Wang WT, Gao ZY, Shi DZ. Effects of Coenzyme Q10 on
Statin-Induced Myopathy: An Updated Meta-Analysis of
Randomized Controlled Trials. J Am Heart Assoc.
2018;7(19):e009835.

"no better than a placebo" Marcoff L, Thompson PD. The
role of coenzyme Q10 in statin-associated myopathy: a
systematic review. J Am Coll Cardiol. 2007;49(23):2231-2237.

"the American College of Cardiology" Vogel JH, Bolling SF,
Costello RB, et al. Integrating complementary medicine into
cardiovascular medicine. J Am Coll Cardiol. 2005;46(1):184-
221.

"American Heart Association" Newman CB, Preiss D, Tobert
JA, et al. Statin Safety and Associated Adverse Events: A
Scientific Statement From the American Heart Association
[published correction appears in Arterioscler Thromb Vasc
Biol. 2019 May;39(5):e158]. Arterioscler Thromb Vasc Biol.
2019;39(2):e38-e81.

"their own scientific journal" Qu H, Guo M, Chai H, et al.
Effects of Coenzyme Q10 on Statin-Induced Myopathy: An
Updated Meta-Analysis of Randomized Controlled Trials.
Journal of the American Heart Association.
2018;7(19):e009835.

"increased chance of developing diabetes" Thompson PD,
Panza G, Zaleski A, Taylor B. Statin-Associated Side Effects. J
Am Coll Cardiol. 2016;67(20):2395-2410.

"the theoretical risk of developing diabetes" Ridker PM, Pradhan A, MacFadyen JG, Libby P, Glynn RJ. Cardiovascular benefits and diabetes risks of statin therapy in primary prevention: an analysis from the JUPITER trial. The Lancet. 2012;380(9841):565-571.

Chapter 2:

"A report on education" Adams KM, Butsch WS, Kohlmeier M. The State of Nutrition Education at US Medical Schools. Journal of Biomedical Education. 2015;2015:1-7.
"When researchers surveyed 646 cardiologists" Devries S, Agatston A, Aggarwal M, et al. A Deficiency of Nutrition Education and Practice in Cardiology. Am J Med. 2017 Nov;130(11):1298-1305..
"More than 40% of Americans are obese" Obesity is a Common, Serious, and Costly Disease. Centers for Disease Control and Prevention. Published November 12, 2021. https://www.cdc.gov/obesity/data/adult.html
"one in five American children" Childhood Obesity Facts. CDC. Published November 12, 2021. https://www.cdc.gov/obesity/data/childhood.html
"the poor only consumed about 1400 calories" Floud R, Fogel RW, Harris B, Hong SC. The Changing Body: Health, Nutrition, and Human Development in the Western World since 1700. Illustrated edition. Cambridge University Press; 2011.
"spent close to 20% of their paychecks on food" Zeballos E & Sinclair W. Average Share of Income Spent on Food in the United States Remained Relatively Steady From 2000 to 2019. USDA. https://www.ers.usda.gov/amber-waves/2020/november/average-share-of-income-spent-on-food-in-the-united-states-remained-relatively-steady-from-

2000-to-2019/

"A dozen eggs in 1919" Allen FL. Only Yesterday. Blue Ribbon Books; 1931.

"incomes have risen roughly 2000%" Statistics of Income From Returns of Net Income for 1920. IRS. https://www.irs.gov/pub/irs-soi/20soirepar.pdf

"plants and vegetables have become less nutritious" Davis DR, Epp MD, Riordan HD. Changes in USDA Food Composition Data for 43 Garden Crops, 1950 to 1999. Journal of the American College of Nutrition. 2004;23(6):669-682.

"may worsen with changing climate conditions" Zhu C, Kobayashi K, Loladze I, et al. Carbon dioxide (CO2) levels this century will alter the protein, micronutrients, and vitamin content of rice grains with potential health consequences for the poorest rice-dependent countries. Science Advances. 2018;4(5).

"people lose roughly the same amount of weight" Rynders CA, Thomas EA, Zaman A, et al. Effectiveness of Intermittent Fasting and Time-Restricted Feeding Compared to Continuous Energy Restriction for Weight Loss. Nutrients. 2019;11(10):2442.

"can reduce inflammatory markers in the blood" Harvie MN, Howell T. Could Intermittent Energy Restriction and Intermittent Fasting Reduce Rates of Cancer in Obese, Overweight, and Normal-Weight Subjects? A Summary of Evidence. Adv Nutr. 2016;7(4):690-705.

"68% were able to stick to the diet" Pannen ST, Maldonado SG, Nonnenmacher T, et al. Adherence and Dietary Composition during Intermittent vs. Continuous Calorie Restriction: Follow-Up Data from a Randomized Controlled Trial in Adults with Overweight or Obesity. Nutrients. 2021; 13(4):1195.

"people tend to lose weight faster with a low-carb diet" Tobias DK, Chen M, Manson JE, et al. Effect of low-fat diet interventions versus other diet interventions on long-term weight change in adults: a systematic review and meta-analysis. Lancet Diabetes Endocrinol. 2015;3(12):968-979.

"better cholesterol and triglyceride numbers on bloodwork" Foster GD, Wyatt HR, Hill JO, et al. A Randomized Trial of a Low-Carbohydrate Diet for Obesity. New England Journal of Medicine. 2003;348(21):2082-2090.

"they find no significant difference in weight loss" Nordmann AJ, Nordmann A, Briel M, et al. Effects of low-carbohydrate vs low-fat diets on weight loss and cardiovascular risk factors: a meta-analysis of randomized controlled trials [published correction appears in Arch Intern Med. 2006 Apr 24;166(8):932]. Arch Intern Med. 2006;166(3):285-293.

"a relatively depressing trend with weight loss" Dansinger ML, Tatsioni A, Wong JB, Chung M, Balk EM. Meta-analysis: the effect of dietary counseling for weight loss. Ann Intern Med. 2007;147(1):41-50.

"age, gender, and socioeconomic status" Varkevisser RDM, van Stralen MM, Kroeze W, Ket JCF, Steenhuis IHM. Determinants of weight loss maintenance: a systematic review. Obes Rev. 2019;20(2):171-211.

"They titled their study Look AHEAD" Group TLAR. The Look AHEAD Study: A Description of the Lifestyle Intervention and the Evidence Supporting It. Obesity. 2006;14(5):737-752.

"At the end of the study" Look AHEAD Research Group, Wing RR, Bolin P, Brancati FL, et al. Cardiovascular effects of intensive lifestyle intervention in type 2 diabetes. N Engl J Med. 2013 Jul 11;369(2):145-54. Epub 2013 Jun 24. Erratum in: N Engl J Med. 2014 May 8;370(19):1866.

"positive findings from the Look AHEAD study" Pi-Sunyer X. The Look AHEAD Trial: A Review and Discussion Of Its Outcomes. Curr Nutr Rep. 2014;3(4):387-391.

"less likely to need hospitalization" Espeland MA, Glick HA, Bertoni A, et al. Impact of an Intensive Lifestyle Intervention on Use and Cost of Medical Services Among Overweight and Obese Adults With Type 2 Diabetes: The Action for Health in Diabetes. Diabetes Care. 2014;37(9):2548-2556.

"The United States Preventive Services Taskforce conducted" Patnode CD, Evans CV, Senger CA, Redmond N, Lin JS. Behavioral Counseling to Promote a Healthful Diet and Physical Activity for Cardiovascular Disease Prevention in Adults Without Known Cardiovascular Disease Risk Factors: Updated Systematic Review for the U.S. Preventive Services Task Force. Rockville (MD): Agency for Healthcare Research and Quality (US); July 2017.

"15 to 20 percent" Wilding JPH, Batterham RL, Davies M, et al. Weight regain and cardiometabolic effects after withdrawal of semaglutide: The STEP 1 trial extension. Diabetes, Obesity and Metabolism. 2022;24(8):1553-1564.

"People who keep healthy foods at home" Paixão C, Dias CM, Jorge R, et al. Successful weight loss maintenance: A systematic review of weight control registries. Obes Rev. 2020;21(5):e13003.

"most descriptions include high consumption of" Trichopoulou, A., Martínez-González, M.A., Tong, T.Y. et al. Definitions and potential health benefits of the Mediterranean diet: views from experts around the world. BMC Med 12, 112 (2014).

"The Mediterranean diet has been linked to" Romagnolo DF, Selmin OI. Mediterranean Diet and Prevention of Chronic Diseases. Nutr Today. 2017;52(5):208-222.

"people could add over ten years" Fadnes LT, Økland JM, Haaland ØA, Johansson KA. Estimating impact of food choices on life expectancy: A modeling study. PLOS Medicine. 2022;19(2):e1003889.

"Cucumbers, cherries, and walnuts all originated from Asia" Lăcătuşu CM, Grigorescu ED, Floria M, Onofriescu A, Mihai BM. The Mediterranean Diet: From an Environment-Driven Food Culture to an Emerging Medical Prescription. Int J Environ Res Public Health. 2019;16(6):942.

Chapter 3

"the majority of the calories" Westerterp KR. Physical activity and physical activity induced energy expenditure in humans: measurement, determinants, and effects. Front Physiol. 2013;4:90. Published 2013 Apr 26.

"what scientists call 'compensatory responses.'" Church TS, Martin CK, Thompson AM, et al. Changes in weight, waist circumference and compensatory responses with different doses of exercise among sedentary, overweight postmenopausal women. PLoS One. 2009;4(2):e4515.

"shows up repeatedly in the scientific literature" Thomas DM, Bouchard C, Church T, et al. Why do individuals not lose more weight from an exercise intervention at a defined dose? An energy balance analysis. Obes Rev. 2012;13(10):835-847.

"with individuals losing less weight than expected" Thivel D, Aucouturier J, Metz L, Morio B, Duché P. Is there spontaneous energy expenditure compensation in response to intensive exercise in obese youth? Pediatr Obes. 2014 Apr;9(2):147-54.

"zero to three percent" Swift DL, McGee JE, Earnest CP, et al. The Effects of Exercise and Physical Activity on Weight Loss and Maintenance. Prog Cardiovasc Dis. 2018 Jul-

Aug;61(2):206-213.

"exercise did seem to augment weight loss" Catenacci VA, Wyatt HR. The role of physical activity in producing and maintaining weight loss. Nat Clin Pract Endocrinol Metab. 2007;3(7):518-529.

"a decreased risk of heart attacks" Yusuf S, Hawken S, Ounpuu S, et al. Effect of potentially modifiable risk factors associated with myocardial infarction in 52 countries (the INTERHEART study): case-control study. Lancet. 2004;364(9438):937-952.

"a smaller risk of developing cancer" Kyu HH, Bachman VF, Alexander LT, et al. Physical activity and risk of breast cancer, colon cancer, diabetes, ischemic heart disease, and ischemic stroke events: systematic review and dose-response meta-analysis for the Global Burden of Disease Study 2013. BMJ. 2016;354:i3857.

"improvements in blood pressure" Whelton SP, Chin A, Xin X, He J. Effect of aerobic exercise on blood pressure: a meta-analysis of randomized, controlled trials. Ann Intern Med. 2002;136(7):493-503.

"a decreased risk of depression" Schuch FB, Vancampfort D, Firth J, et al. Physical Activity and Incident Depression: A Meta-Analysis of Prospective Cohort Studies. Am J Psychiatry. 2018;175(7):631-648.

"routine exercise and increased physical fitness" Myers J, Kaykha A, George S, et al. Fitness versus physical activity patterns in predicting mortality in men. Am J Med. 2004 Dec 15;117(12):912-8.

"have been linked to decreased mortality" Kodama S, Saito K, Tanaka S, et al. Cardiorespiratory fitness as a quantitative predictor of all-cause mortality and cardiovascular events in healthy men and women: a meta-analysis. JAMA.

2009;301(19):2024-2035.

"Even short bouts of exercise" Saint-Maurice PF, Troiano RP, Matthews CE, et al. Moderate-to-Vigorous Physical Activity and All-Cause Mortality: Do Bouts Matter? Journal of the American Heart Association. 2018;7:e007678.

"more intense forms of physical activity" Hooshmand Moghadam B, Golestani F, Bagheri R, et al. The Effects of High-Intensity Interval Training vs. Moderate-Intensity Continuous Training on Inflammatory Markers, Body Composition, and Physical Fitness in Overweight/Obese Survivors of Breast Cancer: A Randomized Controlled Clinical Trial. Cancers (Basel). 2021;13(17):4386. Published 2021 Aug 30.

"Physical Activity Guidelines for Americans" Piercy KL, Troiano RP, Ballard RM, et al. The Physical Activity Guidelines for Americans. JAMA. 2018;320(19):2020-2028.

"increasing physical activity past the minimum recommended" Arem H, Moore SC, Patel A, et al. Leisure time physical activity and mortality: a detailed pooled analysis of the dose-response relationship. JAMA Intern Med. 2015;175(6):959-967.

"individuals who walked just 15 minutes a day" Wen CP, Wai JP, Tsai MK, et al. Minimum amount of physical activity for reduced mortality and extended life expectancy: a prospective cohort study. Lancet. 2011;378(9798):1244-1253.

"Another study on joggers" Schnohr P, O'Keefe JH, Marott JL, Lange P, Jensen GB. Dose of jogging and long-term mortality: the Copenhagen City Heart Study. J Am Coll Cardiol. 2015;65(5):411-419.

"may be a more efficient form" Mendes R, Sousa N, Themudo-Barata JL, Reis VM. High-Intensity Interval Training Versus Moderate-Intensity Continuous Training in Middle-Aged and Older Patients with Type 2 Diabetes: A Randomized

Controlled Crossover Trial of the Acute Effects of Treadmill Walking on Glycemic Control. Int J Environ Res Public Health. 2019 Oct 28;16(21):4163.

"less total time exercising" García-Pinillos F, Laredo-Aguilera JA, Muñoz-Jiménez M, Latorre-Román PA. Effects of 12-Week Concurrent High-Intensity Interval Strength and Endurance Training Program on Physical Performance in Healthy Older People. J Strength Cond Res. 2019 May;33(5):1445-1452.

"the largest mortality benefit was observed in individuals" Stamatakis E, Lee IM, Bennie J, et al. Does Strength-Promoting Exercise Confer Unique Health Benefits? A Pooled Analysis of Data on 11 Population Cohorts With All-Cause, Cancer, and Cardiovascular Mortality Endpoints. Am J Epidemiol. 2018;187(5):1102-1112.

"when elderly women were randomized" Bischoff-Ferrari HA, Vellas B, Rizzoli R, et al. Effect of Vitamin D Supplementation, Omega-3 Fatty Acid Supplementation, or a Strength-Training Exercise Program on Clinical Outcomes in Older Adults: The DO-HEALTH Randomized Clinical Trial. JAMA. 2020;324(18):1855-1868.

"strength training helps build muscle while burning fat" Schmitz KH, Jensen MD, Kugler KC, Jeffery RW, Leon AS. Strength training for obesity prevention in midlife women. Int J Obes Relat Metab Disord. 2003;27(3):326-333.

"individuals randomized to strength training" Strasser B, Siebert U, Schobersberger W. Resistance training in the treatment of the metabolic syndrome: a systematic review and meta-analysis of the effect of resistance training on metabolic clustering in patients with abnormal glucose metabolism. Sports Med. 2010;40(5):397-415.

"BMIs in the normal weight category" Bhaskaran K, Dos-

Santos-Silva I, Leon DA, Douglas IJ, Smeeth L. Association of BMI with overall and cause-specific mortality: a population-based cohort study of 3·6 million adults in the UK. Lancet Diabetes Endocrinol. 2018;6(12):944-953.

"obese but fit individuals can live just as long" Barry VW, Baruth M, Beets MW, et al. Fitness vs. fatness on all-cause mortality: a meta-analysis. Prog Cardiovasc Dis. 2014;56(4):382-390.

"Some experts have proposed" Qiao Q, Nyamdorj R. Is the association of type II diabetes with waist circumference or waist-to-hip ratio stronger than that with body mass index?. Eur J Clin Nutr. 2010;64(1):30-34.

"These methods show some promise" Venkatrao M, Nagarathna R, Patil SS, et al. A composite of BMI and waist circumference may be a better obesity metric in Indians with high risk for type 2 diabetes: An analysis of NMB-2017, a nationwide cross-sectional study. Diabetes Res Clin Pract. 2020;161:108037.

Chapter 4

"patients end up sleeping considerably less" Yoder JC, Staisiunas PG, Meltzer DO, Knutson KL, Arora VM. Noise and sleep among adult medical inpatients: far from a quiet night. Arch Intern Med. 2012;172(1):68-70.

"patients only slept 5.5 hours a night" Adachi M, Staisiunas PG, Knutson KL, Beveridge C, Meltzer DO, Arora VM. Perceived control and sleep in hospitalized older adults: A sound hypothesis?: Sleep in Hospitalized Adults. J Hosp Med. 2013;8(4):184-190.

"experts from the American Academy of Sleep Medicine" Watson NF, Badr MS, Belenky G, et al. Recommended Amount of Sleep for a Healthy Adult: A Joint Consensus

Statement of the American Academy of Sleep Medicine and Sleep Research Society. Sleep. 2015;38(6):843-844.

"Melatonin is a hormone that helps regulate" Zawilska JB, Skene DJ, Arendt J. Physiology and pharmacology of melatonin in relation to biological rhythms. Pharmacol Rep. 2009;61(3):383-410.

"melatonin helped people fall asleep seven minutes faster" Ferracioli-Oda E, Qawasmi A, Bloch MH. Meta-analysis: melatonin for the treatment of primary sleep disorders. PLoS One. 2013;8(5):e63773.

"The Centers for Disease Control report that 35% of Americans" Data and Statistics - Sleep and Sleep Disorders. CDC. Published September 13, 2021. https://www.cdc.gov/sleep/data_statistics.html

"more Americans sleep less than six hours" Knutson KL, Van Cauter E, Rathouz PJ, DeLeire T, Lauderdale DS. Trends in the prevalence of short sleepers in the USA: 1975-2006. Sleep. 2010;33(1):37-45.

"people tend to do worse on cognitive tasks" Belenky G, Wesensten NJ, Thorne DR, et al. Patterns of performance degradation and restoration during sleep restriction and subsequent recovery: a sleep dose-response study. J Sleep Res. 2003;12(1):1-12.

"genetically predisposed to function better on limited sleep" Kuna ST, Maislin G, Pack FM, et al. Heritability of performance deficit accumulation during acute sleep deprivation in twins. Sleep. 2012;35(9):1223-1233.

"33% more likely to have been in an accident" Gottlieb DJ, Ellenbogen JM, Bianchi MT, Czeisler CA. Sleep deficiency and motor vehicle crash risk in the general population: a prospective cohort study. BMC Med. 2018;16(1):44.

"three times as likely to get sick" Cohen S, Doyle WJ, Alper

CM, Janicki-Deverts D, Turner RB. Sleep habits and susceptibility to the common cold. Arch Intern Med. 2009;169(1):62-67.

"20% higher risk of a heart attack" Daghlas I, Dashti HS, Lane J, et al. Sleep Duration and Myocardial Infarction. J Am Coll Cardiol. 2019;74(10):1304-1314.

"Researchers have found benefits of naps" Ruggiero JS, Redeker NS. Effects of napping on sleepiness and sleep-related performance deficits in night-shift workers: a systematic review. Biol Res Nurs. 2014;16(2):134-142.

"sleep inertia, defined as a period of drowsiness" Milner CE, Cote KA. Benefits of napping in healthy adults: impact of nap length, time of day, age, and experience with napping. J Sleep Res. 2009;18(2):272-281.

"Americans report that their naps are a full hour long" 2008 Sleep, Performance and the Workplace. Sleep Foundation. Published October 19, 2018. https://www.sleepfoundation.org/professionals/sleep-americar-polls/2008-sleep-performance-and-workplace

"study subjects who had been chronically sleep restricted" Smith MG, Wusk GC, Nasrini J, et al. Effects of six weeks of chronic sleep restriction with weekend recovery on cognitive performance and wellbeing in high-performing adults. Sleep. 2021;44(8)

"Thomas Edison purported to only sleep four or five hours" Runes DD. The Diary and Sundry Observations of Thomas A. Edison. Philosophical Library; 2007.

"Buckminster Fuller claimed to work" Science: Dymaxion Sleep. Time. Published online October 11, 1943. http://content.time.com/time/subscriber/article/0,33009,774680,00.html

"when sleep scientists reviewed studies on polyphasic sleeping"

Weaver MD, Sletten TL, Foster RG, et al. Adverse impact of polyphasic sleep patterns in humans: Report of the National Sleep Foundation sleep timing and variability consensus panel. Sleep Health. 2021;7(3):293-302.

"Sleep hygiene focuses on setting ourselves up" Sleep Hygiene Tips - Sleep and Sleep Disorders. CDC. Published February 13, 2019. https://www.cdc.gov/sleep/about_sleep/sleep_hygiene.html

"individuals who exercised reported better sleep" Alarcón-Gómez J, Chulvi-Medrano I, Martin-Rivera F, Calatayud J. Effect of High-Intensity Interval Training on Quality of Life, Sleep Quality, Exercise Motivation and Enjoyment in Sedentary People with Type 1 Diabetes Mellitus. Int J Environ Res Public Health. 2021;18(23):12612.

"A separate study examined nursing home residents" Alessi CA, Martin JL, Webber AP, Cynthia Kim E, Harker JO, Josephson KR. Randomized, controlled trial of a nonpharmacological intervention to improve abnormal sleep/wake patterns in nursing home residents. J Am Geriatr Soc. 2005;53(5):803-810.

"some sleep researchers have noticed large discrepancies" Irish LA, Kline CE, Gunn HE, Buysse DJ, Hall MH. The Role of Sleep Hygiene in Promoting Public Health: A Review of Empirical Evidence. Sleep medicine reviews. 2015;22:23.

"naps actually have little impact on nighttime sleep" Pilcher JJ, Michalowski KR, Carrigan RD. The prevalence of daytime napping and its relationship to nighttime sleep. Behav Med. 2001;27(2):71-76.

"have not always found increases in total sleep" Bonnet MH, Alter J. Effects of irregular versus regular sleep schedules on performance, mood and body temperature. Biol Psychol. 1982;14(3-4):287-296.

"Temperature changes of as little" Raymann RJ, Swaab DF, Van Someren EJ. Skin deep: enhanced sleep depth by cutaneous temperature manipulation. Brain. 2008 Feb;131(Pt 2):500-13.

"Many experts claim that a bedroom" The Best Temperature for Sleep. Cleveland Clinic. Published November 16, 2021. https://health.clevelandclinic.org/what-is-the-ideal-sleeping-temperature-for-my-bedroom/

"This therapy, called Cognitive Behavioral Therapy for Insomnia" McCurry SM, Logsdon RG, Teri L, Vitiello MV. Evidence-based psychological treatments for insomnia in older adults. Psychol Aging. 2007;22(1):18-27.

"subjects randomly assigned to CBTI" Drake CL, Kalmbach DA, Arnedt JT, et al. Treating chronic insomnia in postmenopausal women: a randomized clinical trial comparing cognitive-behavioral therapy for insomnia, sleep restriction therapy, and sleep hygiene education. Sleep. 2019;42(2).

"Perhaps that is why weighted blankets" Ekholm B, Spulber S, Adler M. A randomized controlled study of weighted chain blankets for insomnia in psychiatric disorders. Journal of Clinical Sleep Medicine : JCSM : Official Publication of the American Academy of Sleep Medicine. 2020;16(9):1567.

"Mindfulness and meditation may play" Rusch HL, Rosario M, Levison LM, et al. The effect of mindfulness meditation on sleep quality: a systematic review and meta-analysis of randomized controlled trials. Ann N Y Acad Sci. 2019 Jun;1445(1):5-16.

Chapter 5

"more than half of Americans" Back, Lower Limb, and Upper Limb Pain Among U.S. Adults, 2019. Centers for Disease

Control and Prevention.

"disseminated tuberculosis" Gibbs D, McGahan BG, Ropper AE, Xu DS. Back Pain: Differential Diagnosis and Management. Neurologic Clinics. 2023;41(1):61-76.

"But when scientists examined" Abdel Shaheed C, Ferreira GE, Dmitritchenko A, et al. The efficacy and safety of paracetamol for pain relief: an overview of systematic reviews. Med J Aust. 2021;214(7):324-331.

"Only 23% of people" Derry S, Wiffen PJ, Moore R, Bendtsen L. Ibuprofen for acute treatment of episodic tension-type headache in adults. Cochrane Database of Systematic Reviews 2015, Issue 7. Art. No.: CD011474.

"morphine and fentanyl" Vahedi HSM, Hajebi H, Vahidi E, Nejati A, Saeedi M. Comparison between intravenous morphine versus fentanyl in acute pain relief in drug abusers with acute limb traumatic injury. World J Emerg Med. 2019;10(1):27-32.

"date back to" Opium Poppy. Drug Enforcement Administration Museum. https://museum.dea.gov/exhibits/online-exhibits/cannabis-coca-and-poppy-natures-addictive-plants/opium-poppy

"Irish physician Francis Rynd" Boysen PG, Patel JH, King AN. Brief History of Opioids in Perioperative and Periprocedural Medicine to Inform the Future. Ochsner J. 2023;23(1):43-49.

"Harrison Anti-Narcotic Act" Lyden J, Binswanger IA. The United States opioid epidemic. Semin Perinatol. 2019;43(3):123-131.

"The CDC Guidelines on prescribing" Dowell D, Ragan KR, Jones CM, Baldwin GT, Chou R. CDC Clinical Practice Guideline for Prescribing Opioids for Pain - United States, 2022. MMWR Recomm Rep. 2022;71(3):1-95.

"opioid-induced hyperalgesia" Guichard L, Hirve A, Demiri M, Martinez V. Opioid-induced Hyperalgesia in Patients With Chronic Pain: A Systematic Review of Published Cases. Clin J Pain. 2021;38(1):49-57.

"rewire our brain chemistry" Laboureyras E, Boujema MB, Mauborgne A, Simmers J, Pohl M, Simonnet G. Fentanyl-induced hyperalgesia and analgesic tolerance in male rats: common underlying mechanisms and prevention by a polyamine deficient diet. Neuropsychopharmacology. 2022;47(2):599-608.

"like a serious bone infection" Iorio ML, Barbour JR. Recurrent digital infections and osteomyelitis in monozygotic twins with congenital analgesia and compulsive onychophagia. J Child Neurol. 2014;29(7):962-964.

"into a class called muscle relaxers" Chang WJ. Muscle Relaxants for Acute and Chronic Pain. Phys Med Rehabil Clin N Am. 2020;31(2):245-254.

"some antidepressant drugs" Finnerup NB, Attal N, Haroutounian S, et al. Pharmacotherapy for neuropathic pain in adults: a systematic review and meta-analysis. Lancet Neurol. 2015;14(2):162-173.

"is now being evaluated" Cohen SP, Bhatia A, Buvanendran A, et al. Consensus Guidelines on the Use of Intravenous Ketamine Infusions for Chronic Pain From the American Society of Regional Anesthesia and Pain Medicine, the American Academy of Pain Medicine, and the American Society of Anesthesiologists. Reg Anesth Pain Med. 2018;43(5):521-546.

"one of its most notable" Capriotti T. Medical Marijuana. Home Healthc Now. 2016;34(1):10-15.

"has been used for thousands" Zhuang Y, Xing JJ, Li J, Zeng BY, Liang FR. History of acupuncture research. Int Rev

Neurobiol. 2013;111:1-23.

"One study compared real acupuncture" Cherkin DC, Sherman KJ, Avins AL, et al. A randomized trial comparing acupuncture, simulated acupuncture, and usual care for chronic low back pain. Arch Intern Med. 2009;169(9):858-866.

"will frequently resolve" Casiano VE, Sarwan G, Dydyk AM, Varacallo M. Back Pain. In: StatPearls. StatPearls Publishing; 2023. http://www.ncbi.nlm.nih.gov/books/NBK538173/

"tend to expect this sort" Espeland A, Baerheim A, Albrektsen G, Korsbrekke K, Larsen JL. Patients' views on importance and usefulness of plain radiography for low back pain. Spine (Phila Pa 1976). 2001;26(12):1356-1363.

"does not improve pain outcomes" Jarvik JG, Gold LS, Comstock BA, et al. Association of early imaging for back pain with clinical outcomes in older adults [published correction appears in JAMA. 2015 May 5;313(17):1758]. JAMA. 2015;313(11):1143-1153.

"a common reason for knee pain" Luvsannyam E, Jain MS, Leitao AR, Maikawa N, Leitao AE. Meniscus Tear: Pathology, Incidence, and Management. Cureus. 14(5):e25121.

"can also be found incidentally" Englund M, Guermazi A, Gale D, et al. Incidental Meniscal Findings on Knee MRI in Middle-Aged and Elderly Persons. New England Journal of Medicine. 2008;359(11):1108-1115.

"there is not great evidence" Katz JN, Brophy RH, Chaisson CE, et al. Surgery versus Physical Therapy for a Meniscal Tear and Osteoarthritis. New England Journal of Medicine. 2013;368(18):1675-1684.

"physical activity is an effective" Rhon DI, Kim M, Asche CV, et al. Cost-effectiveness of Physical Therapy vs Intra-articular Glucocorticoid Injection for Knee Osteoarthritis: A Secondary Analysis From a Randomized Clinical Trial. JAMA Netw

Open. 2022;5(1):e2142709. Published 2022 Jan 4.

"Guidelines published by the American College of Physicians" Qaseem A, Wilt TJ, McLean RM, Forciea MA. Noninvasive Treatments for Acute, Subacute, and Chronic Low Back Pain: A Clinical Practice Guideline From the American College of Physicians. Ann Intern Med. 2017;166(7):514-530.

"Emergency room doctors are taught" Chang CH, Holmes JF, Mower WR, Panacek EA. Distracting injuries in patients with vertebral injuries. J Emerg Med. 2005;28(2):147-152.

<u>Chapter 6</u>

"In 1911, explorers Douglas Mawson" Shearman DJ. Vitamin A and Sir Douglas Mawson. Br Med J. 1978;1(6108):283-285.

"there is some controversy on the topic" Carrington-Smith D. Mawson and Mertz: a re-evaluation of their ill-fated mapping journey during the 1911–1914 Australasian Antarctic Expedition. Med J Aust. 2005;183(11).

"The word vitamin itself" Spedding S. Vitamins are more Funky than Casimir thought. Australas Med J. 2013;6(2):104-106.

"it could cause a violent sickness" Rodahl K, Moore T. The vitamin A content and toxicity of bear and seal liver. Biochemical Journal. 1943;37(2):166.

"In addition to weakening the immune system" Hall JA, Grainger JR, Spencer SP, Belkaid Y. The role of retinoic acid in tolerance and immunity. Immunity. 2011;35(1):13-22.

"The idea of treating vision impairments" Wolf G. A History of Vitamin A and Retinoids. The FASEB Journal. 1996;10(9):1102-1107.

"Vitamin A supplementation is still used" Early neonatal vitamin A supplementation and infant mortality: an individual participant data meta-analysis of randomised controlled trials.

Arch Dis Child. 2019;104(3):217-226.

"About 30% of Americans are estimated" Bailey RL, Gahche JJ, Lentino CV, et al. Dietary supplement use in the United States, 2003-2006. J Nutr. 2011 Feb;141(2):261-6.

"Well, one study showed that" Age-Related Eye Disease Study Research Group. A randomized, placebo-controlled, clinical trial of high-dose supplementation with vitamins C and E, beta carotene, and zinc for age-related macular degeneration and vision loss: AREDS report no. 8. Arch Ophthalmol. 2001 Oct;119(10):1417-36. Erratum in: Arch Ophthalmol. 2008 Sep;126(9):1251.

"Of course, a different formulation of the supplement" Age-Related Eye Disease Study 2 Research Group. Lutein + zeaxanthin and omega-3 fatty acids for age-related macular degeneration: the Age-Related Eye Disease Study 2 (AREDS2) randomized clinical trial. JAMA. 2013 May 15;309(19):2005-15. Erratum in: JAMA. 2013 Jul 10;310(2):208.

"two other studies showed" Omenn GS, Goodman GE, Thornquist MD, et al. Effects of a combination of beta carotene and vitamin A on lung cancer and cardiovascular disease. N Engl J Med. 1996;334(18):1150-1155.

"an association between vitamin A supplementation" Alpha-Tocopherol, Beta Carotene Cancer Prevention Study Group. The effect of vitamin E and beta carotene on the incidence of lung cancer and other cancers in male smokers. N Engl J Med. 1994;330(15):1029-1035.

"an increased risk of osteoporosis and fracture" Melhus H, Michaëlsson K, Kindmark A, et al. Excessive dietary intake of vitamin A is associated with reduced bone mineral density and increased risk for hip fracture. Ann Intern Med. 1998;129(10):770-778.

"the B vitamins are water-soluble" Kennedy DO. B Vitamins

and the Brain: Mechanisms, Dose and Efficacy--A Review. Nutrients. 2016;8(2):68. Published 2016 Jan 27.

"Deficiencies in B vitamins are linked to" Mikkelsen K, Apostolopoulos V. B Vitamins and Ageing. Subcell Biochem. 2018;90:451-470.

"studies still show that plenty of" Roust LR, DiBaise JK. . Nutrient deficiencies prior to bariatric surgery. Current Opinion in Clinical Nutrition and Metabolic Care. 2017; 20 (2): 138-144.

"Americans have B vitamin deficiencies" Allen LH. How common is vitamin B-12 deficiency?. Am J Clin Nutr. 2009;89(2):693S-6S.

"vitamin B2, also known as riboflavin" Takata Y, Cai Q, Beeghly-Fadiel A, et al. Dietary B vitamin and methionine intakes and lung cancer risk among female never smokers in China. Cancer Causes Control. 2012;23(12):1965-1975.

"increased levels of vitamin B6" Hartman TJ, Woodson K, Stolzenberg-Solomon R, et al. Association of the B-vitamins pyridoxal 5'-phosphate (B(6)), B(12), and folate with lung cancer risk in older men. Am J Epidemiol. 2001;153(7):688-694.

"an analysis of 18 different studies" Zhang, Sui-Liang MDa; Chen, Ting-Song MDb; Ma, Chen-Yun MDc, et al. Effect of vitamin B supplementation on cancer incidence, death due to cancer, and total mortality, Medicine: August 2016 - Volume 95 - Issue 31 - p e3485

"Captain James Cook tried and failed" Stubbs BJ. Captain Cook's beer: the antiscorbutic use of malt and beer in late 18th century sea voyages. Asia Pac J Clin Nutr. 2003;12(2):129-137.

"Scientists have repeatedly questioned" Cerullo G, Negro M, Parimbelli M, et al. The Long History of Vitamin C: From Prevention of the Common Cold to Potential Aid in the

Treatment of COVID-19. Front Immunol. 2020;11:574029.
"the public perception of vitamin C" Duerbeck NB, Dowling DD, Duerbeck JM. Vitamin C. Obstetrical & Gynecological Survey. 2016; 71 (3): 187-193.
"no effect on the risk of stroke" Ascherio A, Rimm EB, Hernán MA, et al. Relation of consumption of vitamin E, vitamin C, and carotenoids to risk for stroke among men in the United States. Ann Intern Med. 1999;130(12):963-970.
"no effect on cancer prevention" Wang L, Sesso HD, Glynn RJ, et al. Vitamin E and C supplementation and risk of cancer in men: posttrial follow-up in the Physicians' Health Study II randomized trial. Am J Clin Nutr. 2014;100(3):915-923.
"no effect on cardiovascular disease" Sesso HD, Buring JE, Christen WG, et al. Vitamins E and C in the prevention of cardiovascular disease in men: the Physicians' Health Study II randomized controlled trial. JAMA. 2008;300(18):2123-2133.
"An analysis of 29 placebo-controlled studies" Hemilä H, Chalker E. Vitamin C for preventing and treating the common cold. Cochrane Database Syst Rev. 2013;2013(1):CD000980.
"One study found an association" Ferraro PM, Curhan GC, Gambaro G, Taylor EN. Total, Dietary, and Supplemental Vitamin C Intake and Risk of Incident Kidney Stones. Am J Kidney Dis. 2016;67(3):400-407.
"A separate case report describes" McLaran CJ, Bett JH, Nye JA, Halliday JW. Congestive cardiomyopathy and haemochromatosis--rapid progression possibly accelerated by excessive ingestion of ascorbic acid. Aust N Z J Med. 1982;12(2):187-188.
"higher levels of vitamin D in the blood" Ginde AA, Mansbach JM, Camargo CA Jr. Association between serum 25-hydroxyvitamin D level and upper respiratory tract infection in the Third National Health and Nutrition Examination Survey.

Arch Intern Med. 2009;169(4):384-390.

"After all, two separate high quality" Murdoch DR, Slow S, Chambers ST, et al. Effect of vitamin D3 supplementation on upper respiratory tract infections in healthy adults: the VIDARIS randomized controlled trial. JAMA. 2012;308(13):1333-1339.

"supplementing vitamin D failed to reduce" Rees JR, Hendricks K, Barry EL, et al. Vitamin D3 supplementation and upper respiratory tract infections in a randomized, controlled trial. Clin Infect Dis. 2013;57(10):1384-1392.

"But the strength of the sunlight also seems to matter" Webb AR, Kline L, Holick MF. Influence of season and latitude on the cutaneous synthesis of vitamin D3: exposure to winter sunlight in Boston and Edmonton will not promote vitamin D3 synthesis in human skin. J Clin Endocrinol Metab. 1988;67(2):373-378.

"vitamin D deficiency is common throughout" Holick MF. Vitamin D deficiency. N Engl J Med. 2007;357(3):266-281.

"An increased risk of cancer" McCullough ML, Zoltick ES, Weinstein SJ, et al. Circulating Vitamin D and Colorectal Cancer Risk: An International Pooling Project of 17 Cohorts. J Natl Cancer Inst. 2019;111(2):158-169.

"an increased chance of developing diabetes" Pittas AG, Chung M, Trikalinos T, et al. Systematic review: Vitamin D and cardiometabolic outcomes. Ann Intern Med. 2010;152(5):307-314.

"an increased risk of inflammatory bowel disease" Del Pinto R, Pietropaoli D, Chandar AK, Ferri C, Cominelli F. Association Between Inflammatory Bowel Disease and Vitamin D Deficiency: A Systematic Review and Meta-analysis. Inflamm Bowel Dis. 2015;21(11):2708-2717.

"has not been convincingly shown to decrease the risk of

cancer" Bjelakovic G, Gluud LL, Nikolova D, et al. Vitamin D supplementation for prevention of cancer in adults. Cochrane Database Syst Rev. 2014;(6):CD007469.

"diabetes, or a whole host" Jorde R, Sneve M, Torjesen P, Figenschau Y. No improvement in cardiovascular risk factors in overweight and obese subjects after supplementation with vitamin D3 for 1 year. J Intern Med. 2010;267(5):462-472.

"Some studies have shown a reduction in mortality" Bjelakovic G, Gluud LL, Nikolova D, et al. Vitamin D supplementation for prevention of mortality in adults. Cochrane Database Syst Rev. 2014;(1):CD007470.

"the United States Preventive Services" Recommendation: Vitamin D Deficiency in Adults: Screening. United States Preventive Services Taskforce. 2021. https://www.uspreventiveservicestaskforce.org/uspstf/recommendation/vitamin-d-deficiency-screening

"they are generally encouraged to treat" Pilz S, Zittermann A, Trummer C, et al. Vitamin D testing and treatment: a narrative review of current evidence. Endocrine Connections. 2019;8(2):R27.

"Vitamin D supplementation might reduce falls" Bordelon P, Ghetu MV, Langan RC. Recognition and Management of Vitamin D Deficiency. AFP. 2009;80(8):841-846.

"and the risk of fractures" Kong SH, Jang HN, Kim JH, Kim SW, Shin CS. Effect of Vitamin D Supplementation on Risk of Fractures and Falls According to Dosage and Interval: A Meta-Analysis. Endocrinol Metab (Seoul). 2022;37(2):344-358.

"supplementation actually could help" Martineau AR, Jolliffe DA, Greenberg L, et al. Vitamin D supplementation to prevent acute respiratory infections: individual participant data meta-analysis. Health Technol Assess. 2019;23(2):1-44.

"Vitamin E is known as an antioxidant" Burton, G W et al. "Is vitamin E the only lipid-soluble, chain-breaking antioxidant in human blood plasma and erythrocyte membranes?." Archives of biochemistry and biophysics vol. 221,1 (1983): 281-90.

"Since free radicals are thought to contribute to cancer" Valko, M et al. "Free radicals, metals and antioxidants in oxidative stress-induced cancer." Chemico-biological interactions vol. 160,1 (2006): 1-40.

"vitamin E supplementation may actually increase" Miller ER 3rd, Pastor-Barriuso R, Dalal D, et al. Meta-analysis: high-dosage vitamin E supplementation may increase all-cause mortality. Ann Intern Med. 2005;142(1):37-46.

"total U.S. sales of supplements are around" Guallar E, Stranges S, Mulrow C, Appel LJ, Miller ER 3rd. Enough is enough: Stop wasting money on vitamin and mineral supplements [published correction appears in Ann Intern Med. 2014 Jan 21;160(2):143]. Ann Intern Med. 2013;159(12):850-851.

"the entire yearly economy of Honduras" World Bank. Gross Domestic Product for Honduras. FRED, Federal Reserve Bank of St. Louis. https://fred.stlouisfed.org/series/MKTGDPHNA646NWDB

"benefits of vitamin supplements" Fortmann SP, Burda BU, Senger CA, Lin JS, Whitlock EP. Vitamin and mineral supplements in the primary prevention of cardiovascular disease and cancer: An updated systematic evidence review for the U.S. Preventive Services Task Force. Ann Intern Med. 2013;159(12):824-834.

"Newborns, however, are frequently deficient" Shearer MJ. Vitamin K metabolism and nutriture. Blood Rev. 1992;6(2):92-104.

"A vitamin K injection given" Sankar MJ, Chandrasekaran A, Kumar P, et al. Vitamin K prophylaxis for prevention of vitamin K deficiency bleeding: a systematic review. Journal of Perinatology. 2016;36(Suppl 1):S29.

"A growing number of parents have been refusing" Marcewicz LH, Clayton J, Maenner M, et al. Parental Refusal of Vitamin K and Neonatal Preventive Services: A Need for Surveillance. Matern Child Health J. 2017;21(5):1079-1084.

"growing mistrust of physicians" Shah SI, Brumberg HL, La Gamma EF. Applying lessons from vaccination hesitancy to address birth dose Vitamin K refusal: Where has the trust gone?. Semin Perinatol. 2020;44(4):151242.

"more likely to refuse" Bernhardt H, Barker D, Reith DM, et al. Declining newborn intramuscular vitamin K prophylaxis predicts subsequent immunisation refusal: A retrospective cohort study. J Paediatr Child Health. 2015;51(9):889-894.

"One explains that vitamin K can" Vitamin K Injection: Uses, Side Effects, Interactions, Pictures, Warnings & Dosing - WebMD. https://www.webmd.com/drugs/2/drug-93625/vitamin-k-injection/details

"The other states that" Vitamin K for newborns. https://www.caringforkids.cps.ca/handouts/pregnancy-and-babies/vitamin-k-for-newborns

"an extraordinarily safe side effect profile" Brousson MA, Klein MC. Controversies surrounding the administration of vitamin K to newborns: a review. CMAJ. 1996;154(3):307-315.

"The vitamin K formulation in" Vitamin K. Office of Dietary Supplements https://ods.od.nih.gov/factsheets/VitaminK-HealthProfessional/

"detailed study has shown no link" Ross JA, Davies SM. Vitamin K prophylaxis and childhood cancer. Med Pediatr Oncol. 2000;34(6):434-437.

"poor transfer of vitamin K through the placenta" Van Winckel M, De Bruyne R, Van De Velde S, Van Biervliet S.

Vitamin K, an update for the paediatrician. Eur J Pediatr. 2009;168(2):127-134.

"fish oil supplementation can improve" Marik PE, Varon J. Omega-3 dietary supplements and the risk of cardiovascular events: a systematic review. Clin Cardiol. 2009;32(7):365-372.

"But leading trials disagree" Abdelhamid AS, Brown TJ, Brainard JS, et al. Omega-3 fatty acids for the primary and secondary prevention of cardiovascular disease. Cochrane Database Syst Rev. 2018;7(7):CD003177.

"Garlic lowers blood glucose" Hou LQ, Liu YH, Zhang YY. Garlic intake lowers fasting blood glucose: meta-analysis of randomized controlled trials. Asia Pac J Clin Nutr. 2015;24(4):575-582.

"gingko may help prevent memory" Butler M, Nelson VA, Davila H, et al. Over-the-Counter Supplement Interventions to Prevent Cognitive Decline, Mild Cognitive Impairment, and Clinical Alzheimer-Type Dementia: A Systematic Review. Ann Intern Med. 2018;168(1):52-62.

"the exact link between fish oil supplements" Šunderić M, Robajac D, Gligorijević N, et al. Is There Something Fishy About Fish Oil? Curr Pharm Des. 2019;25(15):1747-1759.

"Proponents argue it can stop both" Salehi B, Mishra AP, Nigam M, et al. Resveratrol: A Double-Edged Sword in Health Benefits. Biomedicines. 2018;6(3):91.

"rodents taking resveratrol are less likely" Carter LG, D'Orazio JA, Pearson KJ. Resveratrol and cancer: focus on in vivo evidence. Endocrine-Related Cancer. 2014;21(3):R209-R225.

"one trial that concluded resveratrol supplementation" Wong RH, Raederstorff D, Howe PR. Acute Resveratrol Consumption Improves Neurovascular Coupling Capacity in Adults with Type 2 Diabetes Mellitus. Nutrients. 2016;8(7):425.

"with a leading resveratrol researcher explaining" Elton,

Catherine. Has Harvard's David Sinclair Found the Fountain of Youth? Boston Magazine. Published October 29, 2019. https://www.bostonmagazine.com/health/2019/10/29/david-sinclair/

"Opposing studies have questioned" Kjær TN, Ornstrup MJ, Poulsen MM, et al. No Beneficial Effects of Resveratrol on the Metabolic Syndrome: A Randomized Placebo-Controlled Clinical Trial. J Clin Endocrinol Metab. 2017;102(5):1642-1651.

"how or even if resveratrol works in humans" Pezzuto JM. Resveratrol: Twenty Years of Growth, Development and Controversy. Biomol Ther (Seoul). 2019;27(1):1-14.

"there is no national recommendation" Office of Dietary Supplements - Multivitamin/mineral Supplements. https://ods.od.nih.gov/factsheets/MVMS-HealthProfessional/

"small beneficial effects" Vyas CM, Manson JE, Sesso HD, et al. Effect of multivitamin-mineral supplementation versus placebo on cognitive function: Results from the clinic sub-cohort of the COSMOS randomized clinical trial and meta-analysis of three cognitive studies within COSMOS. The American Journal of Clinical Nutrition. 2024;0(0).

"similar effectiveness against depression" St. John's Wort - The Perfect Antidepressant, If You're German. Discover Magazine. Published July 31 2009. https://www.discovermagazine.com/mind/st-johns-wort-the-perfect-antidepressant-if-youre-german

Chapter 7

"the FDA does not approve supplements" Questions and Answers on Dietary Supplements. FDA. Published online June 9, 2020. https://www.fda.gov/food/information-consumers-using-dietary-supplements/questions-and-answers-dietary-supplements

"zero grams of sugar" Tic Tac. https://www.tictac.com/us/en/faq/

"although they did write a strongly worded letter" Nutrition C for FS and A. Guidance for Industry and FDA: Dear Manufacturer Letter Regarding Sugar Free Claims. U.S. Food and Drug Administration. Published September 20, 2021. https://www.fda.gov/regulatory-information/search-fda-guidance-documents/guidance-industry-and-fda-dear-manufacturer-letter-regarding-sugar-free-claims

"When scientists studied the procedure against" Firanescu CE, Vries J de, Lodder P, et al. Vertebroplasty versus sham procedure for painful acute osteoporotic vertebral compression fractures (VERTOS IV): randomised sham controlled clinical trial. BMJ. 2018;361:k1551.

"there was no difference between the sham" Wali AR, Martin JR, Rennert R, et al. Vertebroplasty for vertebral compression fractures: Placebo or effective?. Surg Neurol Int. 2017;8:81.

"some people still argue" Roux C, Cortet B, Bousson V, Thomas T. Vertebroplasty for osteoporotic vertebral fracture. RMD Open. 2021;7(2):e001655.

"can lead to an increased risk of dying" Arima H, Barzi F, Chalmers J. Mortality patterns in hypertension. J Hypertens. 2011;29 Suppl 1:S3-S7.

"it did not help patients avoid" Carlberg B, Samuelsson O, Lindholm LH. Atenolol in hypertension: is it a wise choice? [published correction appears in Lancet. 2005 Feb 19;365(9460):656]. Lancet. 2004;364(9446):1684-1689.

"through a blinded, randomized-controlled trial" Umscheid CA, Margolis DJ, Grossman CE. Key concepts of clinical trials: a narrative review. Postgrad Med. 2011;123(5):194-204.

"But even randomized-controlled trials" Ioannidis JP. Why most published research findings are false. PLoS Med. 2005;2(8):e124.

"loose regulations around the marketing" Starr RR. Too little, too late: ineffective regulation of dietary supplements in the United States. Am J Public Health. 2015;105(3):478-485.

"Independent tests have shown" Syal R. Revealed: many common omega-3 fish oil supplements are 'rancid.' The Guardian. Published January 17, 2022. https://www.theguardian.com/environment/2022/jan/17/revealed-many-common-omega-3-fish-oil-supplements-are-rancid.

"have been found to contain" Cohen PA, Travis JC, Vanhee C, Ohana D, Venhuis BJ. Nine prohibited stimulants found in sports and weight loss supplements: deterenol, phenpromethamine (Vonedrine), oxilofrine, octodrine, beta-methylphenylethylamine (BMPEA), 1,3-dimethylamylamine (1,3-DMAA), 1,4-dimethylamylamine (1,4-DMAA), 1,3-dimethylbutylamine (1,3-DMBA) and higenamine. Clinical Toxicology. 2021;59(11):975-981.

"Only the United States and New Zealand allow" Ventola CL. Direct-to-Consumer Pharmaceutical Advertising: Therapeutic or Toxic? Pharmacy and Therapeutics. 2011;36(10):669.

"25% of American adults" Levine DM, Linder JA, Landon BE. Characteristics of Americans With Primary Care and Changes Over Time, 2002-2015. JAMA Internal Medicine. 2020;180(3):463-466.

"helped battle AIDS" The History of FDA's Role in Preventing the Spread of HIV/AIDS. FDA. Published online March 25, 2021. https://www.fda.gov/about-fda/fda-history-exhibits/history-fdas-role-preventing-spread-hivaids

"In 2013, researchers examined" Prasad V, Vandross A, Toomey C, et al. A decade of reversal: an analysis of 146 contradicted medical practices. Mayo Clin Proc. 2013;88(8):790-798.

"Conducting more high-quality" Prasad V, Cifu A. Ending Medical Reversal: Improving Outcomes, Saving Lives. Johns Hopkins University Press; 2015.

"rural African American men with longstanding" Brandt, Allan M. 1978. "Racism and research: The case of the Tuskegee Syphilis study." The Hastings Center Report 8(6): 21-29.

"Trials must be rigorously reviewed" Pech C, Cob N, Cejka JT. Understanding institutional review boards: practical guidance to the IRB review process. Nutr Clin Pract. 2007;22(6):618-628.

Chapter 8

"reduce symptoms by 4% over the course" Taverner D, Latte J. Nasal decongestants for the common cold. Cochrane Database Syst Rev. 2007;(1):CD001953.

"evidence for common anti-cough treatments" Smith SM, Schroeder K, Fahey T. Over-the-counter (OTC) medications for acute cough in children and adults in community settings. Cochrane Database Syst Rev. 2014;2014(11):CD001831.

"Zinc preparations have been shown" Hemilä H. Zinc lozenges may shorten the duration of colds: a systematic review. Open Respir Med J. 2011;5:51-58.

"side effects such as taste changes" Science M, Johnstone J, Roth DE, Guyatt G, Loeb M. Zinc for the treatment of the common cold: a systematic review and meta-analysis of randomized controlled trials. CMAJ. 2012;184(10):E551-E561.

"permanent loss of smell" Harris G. F.D.A. Warns Against Use of Popular Cold Remedy. The New York Times. https://www.nytimes.com/2009/06/17/health/policy/17nasa l.html. Published June 17, 2009.

"a shocking 46% of patients" Silverman M, Povitz M, Sontrop JM, et al. Antibiotic Prescribing for Nonbacterial Acute Upper Respiratory Infections in Elderly Persons. Ann Intern Med. 2017;166(11):765-774.

"no clinical benefit to the patient" Kenealy T, Arroll B. Antibiotics for the common cold and acute purulent rhinitis. Cochrane Database Syst Rev. 2013;2013(6):CD000247.

"may not improve cold symptoms" Little P, Moore M, Kelly J, et al. Ibuprofen, paracetamol, and steam for patients with respiratory tract infections in primary care: pragmatic randomised factorial trial. BMJ. 2013;347:f6041.

"A large review of oseltamivir studies" Jefferson T, Jones M, Doshi P, et al. Oseltamivir for influenza in adults and children: systematic review of clinical study reports and summary of regulatory comments. BMJ. 2014;348:g2545.

"without any benefit" Fry AM, Goswami D, Nahar K, et al. Efficacy of oseltamivir treatment started within 5 days of symptom onset to reduce influenza illness duration and virus shedding in an urban setting in Bangladesh: a randomised placebo-controlled trial. Lancet Infect Dis. 2014;14(2):109-118.

"One researcher tried to determine" Valtin H. "Drink at least eight glasses of water a day." Really? Is there scientific evidence for "8 x 8"?. Am J Physiol Regul Integr Comp Physiol. 2002;283(5):R993-R1004.

"The American Heart Association suggests" The American Heart Association. Walking 101. https://www.heart.org/idc/groups/heart-public/@wcm/@fc/documents/downloadable/ucm_463348.pdf

"used to increase physical activity" Schneider PL, Bassett DR Jr, Thompson DL, Pronk NP, Bielak KM. Effects of a 10,000 steps per day goal in overweight adults. Am J Health Promot.

2006;21(2):85-89.

"When pedometers became popular" Reynolds G. Do We Really Need to Take 10,000 Steps a Day for Our Health? The New York Times. https://www.nytimes.com/2021/07/06/well/move/10000-steps-health.html. Published July 6, 2021.

"barely averaged 5,000 steps a day" Bassett DRJ, Wyatt HR, Thompson H, Peters JC, Hill JO. Pedometer-Measured Physical Activity and Health Behaviors in U.S. Adults. Medicine & Science in Sports & Exercise. 2010;42(10):1819-1825.

"the less likely they were to die" Saint-Maurice PF, Troiano RP, Bassett DR Jr, et al. Association of Daily Step Count and Step Intensity With Mortality Among US Adults. JAMA. 2020;323(12):1151-1160.

"tracking one's daily steps leads" Chaudhry UAR, Wahlich C, Fortescue R, et al. The effects of step-count monitoring interventions on physical activity: systematic review and meta-analysis of community-based randomised controlled trials in adults. Int J Behav Nutr Phys Act. 2020;17(1):129.

"women averaging just 4,400 steps" Lee IM, Shiroma EJ, Kamada M, et al. Association of Step Volume and Intensity With All-Cause Mortality in Older Women. JAMA Intern Med. 2019;179(8):1105-1112.

"stretching has been shown to increase" Thomas E, Bianco A, Paoli A, Palma A. The Relation Between Stretching Typology and Stretching Duration: The Effects on Range of Motion. Int J Sports Med. 2018;39(4):243-254.

"slightly decreased performance on average" Behm DG, Blazevich AJ, Kay AD, McHugh M. Acute effects of muscle stretching on physical performance, range of motion, and injury incidence in healthy active individuals: a systematic review. Appl Physiol Nutr Metab. 2016;41(1):1-11.

"acknowledged that some studies showed" Behm DG, Chaouachi A. A review of the acute effects of static and dynamic stretching on performance. Eur J Appl Physiol. 2011;111(11):2633-2651.

"Adding to the controversy" Yeung SS, Yeung EW, Gillespie LD. Interventions for preventing lower limb soft-tissue running injuries. Cochrane Database Syst Rev. 2011;(7):CD001256.

"does not reduce the risk" Cheung K, Hume PA, Maxwell L. Delayed Onset Muscle Soreness. Sports Med. 2003;33(2):145-164.

"Berries have been shown to" Kowalska K, Olejnik A. Current evidence on the health-beneficial effects of berry fruits in the prevention and treatment of metabolic syndrome. Curr Opin Clin Nutr Metab Care. 2016;19(6):446-452.

"blueberries are commonly listed as a superfood" van den Driessche JJ, Plat J, Mensink RP. Effects of superfoods on risk factors of metabolic syndrome: a systematic review of human intervention trials. Food Funct. 2018;9(4):1944-1966.

"unclear why kale is declared superior" Šamec D, Urlić B, Salopek-Sondi B. Kale (Brassica oleracea var. acephala) as a superfood: Review of the scientific evidence behind the statement. Crit Rev Food Sci Nutr. 2019;59(15):2411-2422.

"wealthier individuals are much more likely" Oude Groeniger J, van Lenthe FJ, Beenackers MA, Kamphuis CB. Does social distinction contribute to socioeconomic inequalities in diet: the case of 'superfoods' consumption. Int J Behav Nutr Phys Act. 2017;14(1):40.

"Thankfully, the U.S. Department of Agriculture" Organic 101: What the USDA Organic Label Means. https://www.usda.gov/media/blog/2012/03/22/organic-101-

what-usda-organic-label-means

"If 95% or more" Are organic foods worth the price? Mayo Clinic. https://www.mayoclinic.org/healthy-lifestyle/nutrition-and-healthy-eating/in-depth/organic-food/art-20043880

"Organic foods do not appear" Smith-Spangler C, Brandeau ML, Hunter GE, et al. Are Organic Foods Safer or Healthier Than Conventional Alternatives? Ann Intern Med. 2012;157(5):348-366.

"contain less pesticide residues" Mie A, Andersen HR, Gunnarsson S, et al. Human health implications of organic food and organic agriculture: a comprehensive review. Environ Health. 2017;16(1):111. Published 2017 Oct 27.

"humans have genetically modified our food" Oliver MJ. Why We Need GMO Crops in Agriculture. Mo Med. 2014;111(6):492-507.

"a strain of rice has been modified" Kramkowska M, Grzelak T, Czyżewska K. Benefits and risks associated with genetically modified food products. Ann Agric Environ Med. 2013;20(3):413-419.

"the possibility for unexpected allergic reactions" Allergy Centre, Hong Kong Sanatorium and Hospital, Happy Valley, Hong Kong, Lee T, Ho H, Leung T. Genetically modified foods and allergy. Hong Kong Med J. Published online May 5, 2017.

"are tested for safety" Nutrition C for FS and A. How GMOs Are Regulated for Food and Plant Safety in the United States. FDA. Published online January 10, 2022. https://www.fda.gov/food/agricultural-biotechnology/how-gmos-are-regulated-food-and-plant-safety-united-states

"there is no evidence that approved GMOs" Food, genetically modified. World Health Organization. https://www.who.int/news-room/questions-and-answers/item/food-genetically-modified

"to decrease the risk of recurrent seizures" Bough KJ, Rho JM. Anticonvulsant mechanisms of the ketogenic diet. Epilepsia. 2007;48(1):43-58.

"could actually increase mortality" Seidelmann SB, Claggett B, Cheng S, et al. Dietary carbohydrate intake and mortality: a prospective cohort study and meta-analysis. Lancet Public Health. 2018;3(9):e419-e428.

"create an unfavorable environment" Weber DD, Aminzadeh-Gohari S, Tulipan J, et al. Ketogenic diet in the treatment of cancer - Where do we stand?. Mol Metab. 2020;33:102-121.

"no strong evidence for the long-term" O'Neill B, Raggi P. The ketogenic diet: Pros and cons. Atherosclerosis. 2020;292:119-126.

"over-hyped and under-researched" Pitt CE. Cutting through the Paleo hype: The evidence for the Palaeolithic diet. Aust Fam Physician. 2016;45(1):35-38.

"The CDC estimates that alcohol" Alcohol-Attributable Deaths, US, By Sex, Excessive Use. CDC. https://nccd.cdc.gov/DPH_ARDI/Default/Report.aspx?T= AAM&P=1A04A664-0244-42C1-91DE- 316F3AF6B447&R=B885BD06-13DF-45CD-8DD8- AA6B178C4ECE&M=32B5FFE7-81D2-43C5-A892- 9B9B3C4246C7&F=&D=

"there is strong evidence that marijuana" Ebbert JO, Scharf EL, Hurt RT. Medical Cannabis. Mayo Clin Proc. 2018;93(12):1842-1847.

"chronic pain affects more than" Goldberg DS, McGee SJ. Pain as a global public health priority. BMC Public Health. 2011;11:770.

"evidence for potential other benefits" Hill KP, Palastro MD. Medical cannabis for the treatment of chronic pain and other disorders: misconceptions and facts. Pol Arch Intern Med. 2017;127(11):785-789.

"can help people with mental health diagnoses" Walsh Z, Gonzalez R, Crosby K, et al. Medical cannabis and mental health: A guided systematic review. Clin Psychol Rev. 2017;51:15-29.

"cough, wheezing, and shortness of breath" Ghasemiesfe M, Ravi D, Vali M, et al. Marijuana Use, Respiratory Symptoms, and Pulmonary Function: A Systematic Review and Meta-analysis. Ann Intern Med. 2018;169(2):106-115.

"an increased risk of heart attack" Mittleman MA, Lewis RA, Maclure M, Sherwood JB, Muller JE. Triggering myocardial infarction by marijuana. Circulation. 2001;103(23):2805-2809.

"a connection between marijuana use and schizophrenia" Gage SH, Hickman M, Zammit S. Association Between Cannabis and Psychosis: Epidemiologic Evidence. Biol Psychiatry. 2016;79(7):549-556.

Chapter 9

"dense collection of Nobel laureates" The University of Chicago Magazine: August 2003. https://magazine.uchicago.edu/0308/campus-news/streets.shtml

"residents' median income is around" Lartey J. "It's totally unfair": Chicago, where the rich live 30 years longer than the poor. The Guardian. https://www.theguardian.com/us-news/2019/jun/23/chicago-latest-news-life-expectancy-rich-poor-inequality. Published June 23, 2019.

"can expect to live to 90" Chicago's lifespan gap: Streeterville residents live to 90. Englewood residents die at 60. Study finds it's the largest divide in the U.S. Chicago Tribune. Published

June 6, 2019.

"The median income in Englewood" Englewood: Community Data Snapshot. Chicago Metropolitan Agency for Planning. Published August 2021. https://www.cmap.illinois.gov/documents/10180/126764/Englewood.pdf

"life expectancy gap" Large Life Expectancy Gaps in U.S. Cities Linked to Racial & Ethnic Segregation by Neighborhood. NYU Langone News. https://nyulangone.org/news/large-life-expectancy-gaps-us-cities-linked-racial-ethnic-segregation-neighborhood

"a homicide rate 10 times greater" Bogira S. Concentrated poverty and homicide in Chicago. Chicago Reader. Published July 26, 2012. http://chicagoreader.com/blogs/concentrated-poverty-and-homicide-in-chicago/

"can stretch out the door" Krumrey Y. Englewood: Critical Care. South Side Weekly. Published June 23, 2021. https://southsideweekly.com/critical-care/

"Lower-quality housing is associated" Pacheco CM, Ciaccio CE, Nazir N, et al. Homes of low-income minority families with asthmatic children have increased condition issues. Allergy Asthma Proc. 2014;35(6):467-474.

"noticeably higher rates of asthma" Gupta RS, Zhang X, Sharp LK, Shannon JJ, Weiss KB. Geographic variability in childhood asthma prevalence in Chicago. J Allergy Clin Immunol. 2008;121(3):639-645.e1.

"Englewood residents struggle to find" Kolak M, Bradley M, Block DR, et al. Urban foodscape trends: Disparities in healthy food access in Chicago, 2007-2014. Health Place. 2018;52:231-239.

"Per capita income in Ecuador" GDP per capita (current US$) – Ecuador. World Bank.

https://data.worldbank.org/country/ecuador?view=chart
"Life expectancy is 77 years" Life expectancy at birth, total
(years) – Ecuador. World Bank.
https://data.worldbank.org/country/ecuador?view=chart
"United States' life expectancy of 79 years" Life expectancy at
birth, total (years) - United States. World Bank.
https://data.worldbank.org/country/united-states?view=chart
"Americans die younger on average" Tikkanen R, Abrams MK.
U.S. Health Care from a Global Perspective, 2019: Higher
Spending, Worse Outcomes? The Commonwealth Fund.
"Americans simply pay a higher sticker price" Anderson GF,
Hussey P, Petrosyan V. It's Still The Prices, Stupid: Why The
US Spends So Much On Health Care, And A Tribute To Uwe
Reinhardt. Health Affairs. 2019;38(1):87-95.
"can cost ten times more" The Astronomical Price of Insulin
Hurts American Families. Published January 6, 2021.
https://www.rand.org/blog/rand-review/2021/01/the-
astronomical-price-of-insulin-hurts-american-families.html
"tried to calculate the value" Shrank WH, Rogstad TL, Parekh
N. Waste in the US Health Care System: Estimated Costs and
Potential for Savings. JAMA. 2019;322(15):1501-1509.
"common models do stand out" Reid T. The Healing of
America: A Global Quest for Better, Cheaper, and Fairer
Health Care. Penguin Books; 2010.
"A classic experiment done by the RAND corporation" Brook
RH, Keeler EB, Lohr KN, et al. The Health Insurance
Experiment: A Classic RAND Study Speaks to the Current
Health Care Reform Debate. RAND Corporation; 2006.
https://www.rand.org/pubs/research_briefs/RB9174.html
"when Oregon expanded Medicaid" Oregon Health Insurance
Experiment. NBER. https://www.nber.org/programs-
projects/projects-and-centers/oregon-health-insurance-

experiment

"does not lead to improved health" Malani A, Holtzmann P, Imai K. Effect of Health Insurance in India: A Randomized Controlled Trial. National Bureau of Economic Research; 2021.

"stretch the rules of the patent protection" Gupta H, Kumar S, Roy SK, Gaud RS. Patent protection strategies. J Pharm Bioallied Sci. 2010;2(1):2-7.

"have started to tie reimbursement payments" Ray JC, Kusumoto F. The transition to value-based care. J Interv Card Electrophysiol. 2016;47(1):61-68.

"capped insulin costs" Putterman S. Biden touts $35 insulin cap, overstates prior average cost. Politifact. https://www.politifact.com/factchecks/2024/apr/02/joe-biden/biden-is-right-about-35-insulin-cap-but-exaggerate/

"The Medicare program helps fund" Medical school enrollments grow, but residency slots haven't kept pace. AAMC. https://www.aamc.org/news-insights/medical-school-enrollments-grow-residency-slots-haven-t-kept-pace

"Primary care doctors tend to make" Medscape Physician Compensation Report 2021: The Recovery Begins. Medscape. https://www.medscape.com/slideshow/2021-compensation-overview-6013761

"which receive special funds to offer" Federally Qualified Health Centers. U.S. Health Resources & Services Administration. Published April 21, 2017. https://www.hrsa.gov/opa/eligibility-and-registration/health-centers/fqhc/index.html

"these taxes have been successful" Powell LM, Leider J. Evaluation of Changes in Beverage Prices and Volume Sold Following the Implementation and Repeal of a Sweetened Beverage Tax in Cook County, Illinois. JAMA Netw Open.

2020;3(12):e2031083.

Chapter 10

"an appalling 74% of American adults" Obesity and Overweight. CDC. Published September 10, 2021. https://www.cdc.gov/nchs/fastats/obesity-overweight.htm
"14% of American adults still smoke" Current Cigarette Smoking Among Adults in the United States. Centers for Disease Control and Prevention. Published December 15, 2020. https://www.cdc.gov/tobacco/data_statistics/fact_sheets/adult_data/cig_smoking/index.htm
"between 60% and 80% of Americans" Sharma KP, Grosse SD, Maciosek MV, et al. Preventing Breast, Cervical, and Colorectal Cancer Deaths: Assessing the Impact of Increased Screening. Prev Chronic Dis. 2020;17:E123.
"reduces the risk of dying from colorectal cancer" Doubeni CA, Corley DA, Quinn VP, et al. Effectiveness of screening colonoscopy in reducing the risk of death from right and left colon cancer: a large community-based study. Gut. 2018;67(2):291-298.
"Roughly 50,000 Americans die" Cancer of the Colon and Rectum - Cancer Stat Facts. SEER. https://seer.cancer.gov/statfacts/html/colorect.html
"pale in comparison to the amount of lives" Leading Causes of Death. CDC. Published January 13, 2022. https://www.cdc.gov/nchs/fastats/leading-causes-of-death.htm
"Task Force gives pancreatic cancer screening" US Preventive

Services Task Force. Screening for Pancreatic Cancer: US Preventive Services Task Force Reaffirmation Recommendation Statement. JAMA. 2019;322(5):438-444.

"about 6% of people have adrenal tumors" Moalem J, Suh I, Duh QY. Incidentaloma. In: Sturgeon C, ed. Endocrine Neoplasia. Cancer Treatment and Research. Springer US; 2010:119-134.

"can help save money overall" Maciosek MV, Coffield AB, Flottemesch TJ, Edwards NM, Solberg LI. Greater Use Of Preventive Services In U.S. Health Care Could Save Lives At Little Or No Cost. Health Affairs. 2010;29(9):1656-1660.

"net cost to the healthcare system" Dabestani NM, Leidner AJ, Seiber EE, et al. A review of the cost-effectiveness of adult influenza vaccination and other preventive services. Prev Med. 2019;126:105734.

"gives prostate cancer screening a 'C' rating" US Preventive Services Task Force. Screening for Prostate Cancer: US Preventive Services Task Force Recommendation Statement. JAMA. 2018;319(18):1901-1913.

"failed to find that screening prevented" Fenton JJ, Weyrich MS, Durbin S, et al. Prostate-Specific Antigen–Based Screening for Prostate Cancer: Evidence Report and Systematic Review for the US Preventive Services Task Force. JAMA. 2018;319(18):1914-1931.

"five out of every 1,000 people died" Decision Aid Tool. American Society of Clinical Oncology; 2012. https://www.asco.org/sites/new-www.asco.org/files/content-files/practice-and-guidelines/documents/2012-psa-pco-decision-aid.pdf

"46 recommendations receiving either" United States Preventive Services Taskforce. https://www.uspreventiveservicestaskforce.org/uspstf/

"would spend 8.6 hours a day" Privett N, Guerrier S. Estimation of the Time Needed to Deliver the 2020 USPSTF Preventive Care Recommendations in Primary Care. Am J Public Health. 2021;111(1):145-149.

"not part of any preventive guidelines" Bloomfield HE, Wilt TJ. Evidence Brief: Role of the Annual Comprehensive Physical Examination in the Asymptomatic Adult. In: VA Evidence Synthesis Program Evidence Briefs. Washington (DC): Department of Veterans Affairs (US); October 2011.

"no specific recommendation for a comprehensive yearly" Artandi MK, Stewart RW. The Outpatient Physical Examination. Med Clin North Am. 2018;102(3):465-473.

"they failed to reduce the risks of disability" Krogsbøll LT, Jørgensen KJ, Larsen CG, Gøtzsche PC. General health checks in adults for reducing morbidity and mortality from disease: Cochrane systematic review and meta-analysis. BMJ. 2012;345:e7191.

"a link between regular outpatient appointments" Shein DM, Stone VE. The Annual Physical: Delivering Value. Am J Med. 2017;130(5):507-508.

Chapter 11

"Around 30 percent of senior citizens" Khezrian M, McNeil CJ, Murray AD, Myint PK. An overview of prevalence, determinants and health outcomes of polypharmacy. Therapeutic Advances in Drug Safety. 2020;11.

"Exercise is one of the best ways" Fransen M, McConnell S, Harmer AR, et al. Exercise for osteoarthritis of the knee: a Cochrane systematic review. Br J Sports Med. 2015;49(24):1554-1557.

"unable to dramatically reduce pain" Messier SP, Mihalko SL,

Legault C, et al. Effects of intensive diet and exercise on knee joint loads, inflammation, and clinical outcomes among overweight and obese adults with knee osteoarthritis: the IDEA randomized clinical trial. JAMA. 2013;310(12):1263-1273.

"Anti-inflammatory medications and" Pavelka K. A comparison of the therapeutic efficacy of diclofenac in osteoarthritis: a systematic review of randomised controlled trials. Curr Med Res Opin. 2012;28(1):163-178.

"about 10% of knee replacements" Bayliss LE, Culliford D, Monk AP, et al. The effect of patient age at intervention on risk of implant revision after total replacement of the hip or knee: a population-based cohort study [published correction appears in Lancet. 2017 Apr 8;389(10077):1398]. Lancet. 2017;389(10077):1424-1430.

"the Boscombe Valley Mystery" Doyle AC. The Complete Sherlock Holmes, Volume I. Barnes & Noble Classics; 2003.

"improved diet and exercise, even in middle" Michel JP, Dreux C, Vacheron A. Healthy ageing: Evidence that improvement is possible at every age. European Geriatric Medicine. 2016;7(4):298-305.

"has a side effect of considerable weight loss" Christou GA, Katsiki N, Blundell J, Fruhbeck G, Kiortsis DN. Semaglutide as a promising antiobesity drug. Obesity Reviews. 2019;20(6):805-815.

"Although around 90% of lung cancers" de Groot P, Munden RF. Lung Cancer Epidemiology, Risk Factors, and Prevention. Radiologic Clinics of North America. 2012;50(5):863-876.

"is a stunning 99 percent" SEER Cancer Statistics Review, 1975-2016. National Cancer Institute. https://seer.cancer.gov/csr/1975_2016/index.html

"Smoking cigarettes likely increased" Jones ME, Schoemaker

MJ, Wright LB, Ashworth A, Swerdlow AJ. Smoking and risk of breast cancer in the Generations Study cohort. Breast Cancer Research. 2017;19(1):118.

"the Harvard Study of Adult Development" Mineo L. Over nearly 80 years, Harvard study has been showing how to live a healthy and happy life. Harvard Gazette. Published April 11, 2017.

"Results from the study show" Vaillant GE, Mukamal K. Successful aging. Am J Psychiatry. 2001;158(6):839-847.

"elderly subjects who engaged" Verghese J, Lipton RB, Katz MJ, et al. Leisure activities and the risk of dementia in the elderly. N Engl J Med. 2003;348(25):2508-2516.

"Another trial used a high-quality" Tennstedt SL, Unverzagt FW. The ACTIVE study: study overview and major findings. J Aging Health. 2013;25(8 Suppl):3S-20S.

"with a higher quantity and quality" Holt-Lunstad J, Smith TB, Layton JB. Social relationships and mortality risk: a meta-analytic review. PLoS Med. 2010;7(7):e1000316. Published 2010 Jul 27.

"After just a few months of volunteering" Fried LP, Carlson MC, Freedman M, et al. A social model for health promotion for an aging population: initial evidence on the Experience Corps model. J Urban Health. 2004;81(1):64-78.

"biological, psychological, and social components" Wade DT, Halligan PW. The biopsychosocial model of illness: a model whose time has come. Clin Rehabil. 2017;31(8):995-1004.

Chapter 12

"Patients who receive CPR on television" Portanova J, Irvine K, Yi JY, Enguidanos S. It isn't like this on TV: Revisiting CPR survival rates depicted on popular TV shows. Resuscitation. 2015;96:148-150.

"patient preferences for their code status differed" Young KA, Wordingham SE, Strand JJ, Roger VL, Dunlay SM. Discordance of Patient-Reported and Clinician-Ordered Resuscitation Status in Patients Hospitalized with Acute Decompensated Heart Failure. Journal of pain and symptom management. 2017;53(4):745.

"many change their minds" Murphy DJ, Burrows D, Santilli S, et al. The Influence of the Probability of Survival on Patients' Preferences Regarding Cardiopulmonary Resuscitation. New England Journal of Medicine. 1994;330(8):545-549.

"only about 10% of patients" Yan S, Gan Y, Jiang N, et al. The global survival rate among adult out-of-hospital cardiac arrest patients who received cardiopulmonary resuscitation: a systematic review and meta-analysis. Critical Care. 2020;24(1):61.

"life expectancy for the healthiest" Oeppen J, Vaupel JW. Broken Limits to Life Expectancy. Science. 2002;296(5570):1029-1031.

"Maternal death rates have fallen" Loudon I. Deaths in childbed from the eighteenth century to 1935. Med Hist. 1986;30(1):1-41.

"lived longer on average" Bannister CA, Holden SE, Jenkins-Jones S, et al. Can people with type 2 diabetes live longer than those without? A comparison of mortality in people initiated with metformin or sulphonylurea monotherapy and matched, non-diabetic controls. Diabetes Obes Metab. 2014;16(11):1165-1173.

"increase the average lifespan of mice and roundworms" Soukas AA, Hao H, Wu L. Metformin as Anti-Aging Therapy: Is It for Everyone? Trends in endocrinology and metabolism: TEM. 2019;30(10):745.

"caloric restriction extends lifespan" Pifferi F, Aujard F.

Caloric restriction, longevity and aging: Recent contributions from human and non-human primate studies. Prog Neuropsychopharmacol Biol Psychiatry. 2019;95:109702.

"argue that we can simply develop drugs" Madeo F, Carmona-Gutierrez D, Hofer SJ, Kroemer G. Caloric Restriction Mimetics against Age-Associated Disease: Targets, Mechanisms, and Therapeutic Potential. Cell Metab. 2019;29(3):592-610.

"Many of America's founding fathers" Founding Fathers. Biography.com. https://www.biography.com/people/groups/founding-fathers

"However, opposing studies note" Stockwell T, Zhao J, Panwar S, Roemer A, Naimi T, Chikritzhs T. Do "Moderate" Drinkers Have Reduced Mortality Risk? A Systematic Review and Meta-Analysis of Alcohol Consumption and All-Cause Mortality. J Stud Alcohol Drugs. 2016;77(2):185-198.

"no level of alcohol consumption is safe" Alcohol and health: all, none, or somewhere in-between? The Lancet Rheumatology. 2023;5(4):e167.

"reports of cardiac arrest survivors" Parnia S, Waller DG, Yeates R, Fenwick P. A qualitative and quantitative study of the incidence, features and aetiology of near death experiences in cardiac arrest survivors. Resuscitation. 2001;48(2):149-156.

"developed an ingenious study protocol" Parnia S, Spearpoint K, de Vos G, et al. AWARE—AWAreness during REsuscitation—A prospective study. Resuscitation. 2014;85(12):1799-1805.

Chapter 13

"Comprehensive dietary changes can spur" Ozemek C, Tiwari S, Sabbahi A, Carbone S, Lavie CJ. Impact of therapeutic lifestyle changes in resistant hypertension. Prog Cardiovasc Dis. 2020;63(1):4-9.

"nearly half of American adults" CDC. Facts About Hypertension. Centers for Disease Control and Prevention. Published September 27, 2021. https://www.cdc.gov/bloodpressure/facts.htm

"An estimated 20 to 30% of prescriptions" Viswanathan M, Golin CE, Jones CD, et al. Interventions to Improve Adherence to Self-administered Medications for Chronic Diseases in the United States. Ann Intern Med. 2012;157(11):785-795.

"One poll found that" Armstrong K, Rose A, Peters N, Long JA, McMurphy S, Shea JA. Distrust of the Health Care System and Self-Reported Health in the United States. J Gen Intern Med. 2006;21(4):292-297.

"patients referred to the Mayo Clinic" Van Such M, Lohr R, Beckman T, Naessens JM. Extent of diagnostic agreement among medical referrals. J Eval Clin Pract. 2017;23(4):870-874.

"tend to delay potentially lifesaving care" Powell W, Richmond J, Mohottige D, Yen I, Joslyn A, Corbie-Smith G. Medical Mistrust, Racism, and Delays in Preventive Health Screening Among African-American Men. Behavioral Medicine. 2019;45(2):102-117.

"a 2016 article in the British Medical Journal" Makary MA, Daniel M. Medical error-the third leading cause of death in the US. BMJ. 2016;353:i2139. Published 2016 May 3.

"if a patient received an antibiotic" Shojania KG, Dixon-Woods M. Estimating deaths due to medical error: the ongoing controversy and why it matters. BMJ Qual Saf. 2017;26(5):423-428.

"Other research, although less frequently cited" Rodwin BA, Bilan VP, Merchant NB, et al. Rate of Preventable Mortality in

Hospitalized Patients: a Systematic Review and Meta-analysis. J Gen Intern Med. 2020;35(7):2099-2106.

"with lawsuits being commonplace" Gawande A. The Malpractice Mess. The New Yorker. Published online November 6, 2005. https://www.newyorker.com/magazine/2005/11/14/the-malpractice-mess

"average over 16 minutes on the computer" Overhage JM, McCallie D. Physician Time Spent Using the Electronic Health Record During Outpatient Encounters: A Descriptive Study. Ann Intern Med. 2020;172(3):169-174.

"A majority of U.S. physicians" West CP, Dyrbye LN, Shanafelt TD. Physician burnout: contributors, consequences and solutions. J Intern Med. 2018;283(6):516-529.

ABOUT THE AUTHOR

Dr. Miksanek is a graduate of the University of Chicago Pritzker School of Medicine. He has been inducted into the Alpha Omega Alpha Honor Medical Society, and his scientific writing has been published in *Annals of Internal Medicine* and *JAMA Network Open*. His research on health care economics has won the Joseph P. Kirsner Research Award for Excellence and the John D. Arnold, MD Scientific Research Prize. This is his first book.

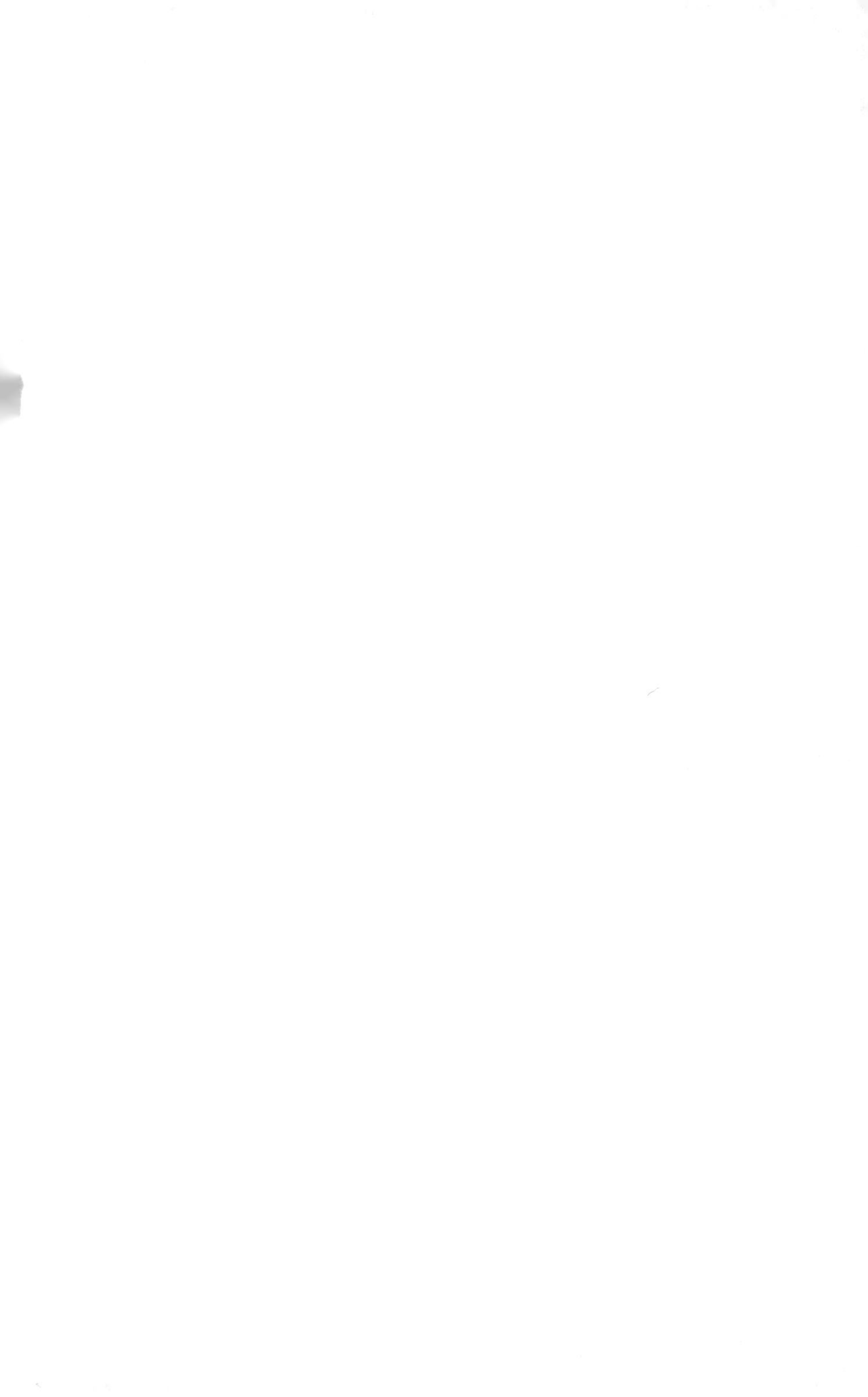